The Ultimate Metabolism Diet

About the Author

Scott Rigden, MD, practices medicine in Chandler, Arizona, where he specializes in weight-loss management (bariatrics) and nutritional approaches to chronic illness. His long-standing professional interest in obesity began with his own weight struggles as a child and teen, when he had to lose 65 pounds. After graduating cum laude from Cornell University, he completed his medical studies at St. Louis University Medical School and the Family Practice residency program at Sparrow Hospital in Lansing, Michigan. During this time, Dr. Rigden published original research on the long-term medical consequences of the small bowel bypass surgery procedure for weight loss.

In addition to maintaining his busy practice, Dr. Rigden has presented many classes and seminars to lay people and fellow professionals on obesity and related topics. He has published numerous articles and is the author of *Take It Off: The Weight Workbook.*

The American Society of Bariatric Physicians honored him as one of 15 recipients in its 50-year history with the designation of Fellow for his excellence in the field of bariatrics. Dr. Rigden also earned the honor of being named HealthComm Researcher of the Year for his work on chronic fatigue syndrome and fibromyalgia. He is a pioneer in the emerging field of functional medicine, a medical discipline that emphasizes the integration of the whole person and nutritional biochemistry. Dr. Rigden received the Institute of Functional Medicine Outstanding Contribution Award. He is a Diplomate and Fellow of the American Board of Family Practice and a Diplomate of the American Board of Bariatric Medicine.

Barbara Schiltz, RN, MS, CN, is a professional nurse. She earned her undergraduate degree in foods and nutrition and her master's degree in nutrition from Bastyr University, located in Seattle, Washington. Since 1996 she has worked as a nutrition consultant and research nurse at the Functional

Medicine Research Center (FMRC) in Gig Harbor, Washington, monitoring patients undergoing clinical trials for diabetes, insulin resistance, and other medical conditions. Her special interest was expressed in her thesis, "The Unique Role of Carbohydrate Metabolism in Regulation of Glycemic Index." Subsequently, she was instrumental in the development of the low-glycemic-index dietary program for the FMRC. Barb frequently lectures and is the coauthor of a number of articles on such topics as managing diabetes and metabolic syndrome with low-glycemic-index diets, and diagnosing and managing food allergies. She is a gourmet cook who enjoys developing healthy recipes and menu ideas.

Ordering
Trade bookstores in the U.S. and Canada please contact:

Publishers Group West
1700 Fourth Street, Berkeley CA 94710
Phone: (800) 788-3123   Fax: (800) 351-5073

Hunter House books are available at bulk discounts
for textbook course adoptions; to qualifying community, health-care,
and government organizations; and for special promotions and fund-raising.
For details please contact:

Special Sales Department
Hunter House Inc., PO Box 2914, Alameda CA 94501-0914
Phone: (510) 865-5282   Fax: (510) 865-4295
E-mail: ordering@hunterhouse.com

Individuals can order our books from most bookstores,
by calling **(800) 266-5592**, or from our website at
www.hunterhouse.com

The Ultimate Metabolism Diet

Eat Right for Your Metabolic Type

Scott Rigden, MD

WITH BARBARA SCHILTZ, RN

Hunter House PUBLISHERS

Hunter House Inc., Publishers
PO Box 2914
Alameda CA 94501-0914

Library of Congress Cataloging-in-Publication Data
Rigden, Scott, 1948-
The ultimate metabolism diet : eat right for your metabolic type / Scott Rigden, Barbara Schiltz. — 1st ed.
p.   cm.
Includes bibliographical references and index.
ISBN-13: 978-0-89793-510-4 (pbk.)
ISBN-10: 0-89793-510-1 (pbk.)
1. Reducing diets. 2. Weight loss. 3. Metabolism—Regulation. 4. Low-fat diet.
I. Schiltz, Barbara. II. Title.
RM222.2.R52 2009
613.2'5—dc22   2008024261

Project Credits

Cover Design	Brian Dittmar Graphic Design
Book Production	John McKercher
Developmental and Copy Editor	Mary Miller
Proofreader	John David Marion
Indexer	Nancy D. Peterson
Editor	Alexandra Mummery
Senior Marketing Associate	Reina Santana
Publicity Intern	Sean Harvey
Production Assistant	Amy Hagelin
Rights Coordinator	Candace Groskreutz
Customer Service Manager	Christina Sverdrup
Order Fulfillment	Washul Lakdhon
Administrator	Theresa Nelson
Computer Support	Peter Eichelberger
Publisher	Kiran S. Rana

Printed and Bound by Bang Printing, Brainerd, Minnesota

Manufactured in the United States of America

9 8 7 6 5 4 3 2 1   First Edition   08 09 10 11 12

Contents

||||||||||||||||||||||||||||||||||||||||||||||||||||||||||||||||||||

Foreword

I have been in the fields of preventive and nutritional medicine for 33 years. I have known Scott Rigden, MD, for 30 of these years. He has always been a "clinician's clinician," providing the best of family medicine to his patients. He is a unique blend of a pragmatic doctor who is concerned more about what improves his patient's health outcome than convention, coupled with the pursuit of what lies at the evolving frontier in health sciences that he can add to his skills.

He is a true expert in metabolic medicine and bariatrics, or the science of weight loss. He has been a leader in the field for more than 25 years, having successfully treated thousands of patients who had failed to be successful in regaining their health through the best efforts of many doctors. He has successfully treated the most difficult of the "walking wounded" type of patient—those with chronic fatigue syndrome, fibromyalgia, and long-term obesity and the attendant effects of insulin resistance, type 2 diabetes, and vascular disease. These are not the type of patients that most doctors would like to build a practice or reputation upon because their traditional outcome is so poor. However, Dr. Rigden has made a reputation of successfully treating these types of patients, resulting in long-term positive health outcomes for them.

Why has he been successful where most doctors have not? In getting to know Dr. Rigden very well over the past three decades, I believe it is a result of two factors. One is his indomitable spirit that coaches the patient to success, and the second is his remarkable program that differs considerably from the "standard of care" that most doctors employ with patients of this type. Dr. Rigden has never "bought in" to the concept that people who gain weight do so solely as a consequence of a lack of self-control and excess calorie consumption. As you will learn in this book, he has taken a larger view of the obesity-fatigue-chronic pain complex than to conclude that it is simply a result of eating too many calories.

It is very interesting that if you explore the medical literature, you will find no data indicating we have increased our per capita intake of calories to a level that accounts for the increase in obesity we have witnessed in the past 30 years. In fact, during this period we have seen lower calorie, low-fat diets and foods being promoted more than ever, but the prevalence of obesity-related health problems continues to increase. Dr. Rigden is on top of the latest research that indicates it is more than just "calories" that are the cause of the problem. In fact, it might be that obesity is the effect and not the cause of the problems we are witnessing today, such as the rising epidemic of type 2 diabetes, sleep apnea, high blood pressure, fatigue, and immune problems.

The calorie is a unit of heat energy and, as such, has "no personality" when it comes to its influence on our metabolism. Recent medical science discoveries are finding that when we eat, we eat more than calories. We actually eat information that comes from the composition of our food. This information is "read" by our genes and alters our metabolism and how we look, act, and feel over years of eating and living a certain way. Our body shape is a reflection of what we eat, how we live, the environment we are exposed to, and the stress we are under. Dr. Rigden approaches his patients with this concept as the principle way with which he develops a personalized program for their needs. The combination of genetic background, lifestyle, diet, and environmental assessment gives rise to a different understanding of the patient than just the evaluation of their calorie intake and their activity patterns.

Our bodies are controlled by complex metabolic processes. The calorie content of our diet is only one small part of what influences how our bodies store or utilize energy. We all know that a person who is overweight looks as if they are storing too much energy in the form of body fat, but they often behave as if they don't have enough energy to get through the day. This "switched metabolism" is a result of more than eating too many calories. Rather, it reflects a complex message that the body is translating from the diet and environment that results in a situation of storage of energy as fat rather than utilization of the energy from food for activity.

This is much more complex than just saying a person has hormone problems. In this book you will learn that this switched metabolism contributes to an alteration in physiological function that results not only in storing body fat, but also has an effect on fatigue, insulin resistance, muscle and joint pain, low energy, and digestive problems. You will learn how Dr. Rigden, like a detective, has pieced this puzzle together during his three decades of dedication to his patients and his pursuit of discovery.

The field of medicine is changing rapidly. What we often thought were "truths" only a few years ago are now frequently found to be incorrect. The primacy of the calorie as the solution to the obesity epidemic is one of those "truths" that is under revision. If it were so simple that reduction of calorie intake could solve all the health problems surrounding obesity, the problem would have been solved long ago with the advent of reduced calorie foods and beverages.

Because food carries information to our genes to tell them how to express themselves, the issue is one of delivering the wrong information to the body. This information that comes from the food, lifestyle, and environment of today then signals to the body to respond by storing calories as fat, producing an inflammatory response, and altering our appetite and digestive function. Dr. Rigden provides not only a detailed explanation of this remarkable change in thinking about the origin of our chronic health problems, but also a detailed program based upon his decades of clinical experience and a plan as to how to use this program in an individualized manner.

The world does not need another diet book. There are already too many of them. In fact, none of the best-selling diet books really deliver on providing long-term health solutions. This book is different. It does not focus on weight as the primary problem, but rather as the result of inappropriate messages the body is receiving. You will learn how to recognize these inappropriate signals and how to change them from messages of alarm to messages of physiological harmony. This book represents a new approach to weight management. It is not a recapitulation of what everyone else has been saying about the topic, opinions that have never demonstrated to be successful. Rather, this book provides a fresh and innovative approach based on the latest discoveries in the health sciences, coupled with Dr. Rigden's 30 years of real clinical successes with difficult patients and his unique approach that you will learn how to apply. The information in this book is groundbreaking. It has the potential to change health and health care if it were understood and applied by medicine. The change in medicine may take years, but for you, the reader, the benefit of Dr. Rigden's experience and expertise is available now. I am pleased that you will be a reader of this book and an ambassador for many others who will benefit from your experience in applying this information successfully in your life.

— Jeffrey Bland, PhD, FACN, FACB
Fellow, American College of Nutrition

Acknowledgments

Some key teachers from early in my medical training who inspired me greatly include Duane Hagen, MD, at St. Louis University Medical School, Dr. Skip Ruth at the E. W. Sparrow Hospital Family Practice Residency Program in Lansing, Michigan, and the late Dr. Evarts Loomis, Hemet, California. I greatly appreciate the editorial assistance provided by Sara Benum. My long-standing colleague and friend, David Brunworth, MD, has patiently read early manuscripts and made helpful suggestions. Many colleagues in the American Society of Bariatric Physicians have helped me become a better bariatrician, and I especially would like to acknowledge the late Peter Lindner, MD, and Robert Stark, MD, for nurturing and encouraging me.

Many colleagues at the Institute for Functional Medicine have taught me much through the years. Contributing author Barb Schiltz has generously shared many ideas that have influenced me and helped my patients. Jeffrey Bland, PhD, has been a constant inspiration to me for the past 28 years and has been my main teacher regarding nutrition and nutritional biochemistry. My clinical staff has provided great support in implementing the ideas in this book at our office in Chandler, Arizona, and I want to acknowledge LaRue Lepetich, Marie Hopper, Evita Quintos, Geri Julin, Lisa Davis, and Tracy Baginski. Last, but not least, I would like to thank my patients for their encouragement and input regarding the book; their success stories have inspired and helped me persist for many years in a difficult and challenging field.

DEDICATION

||||||||||||||||||||||||||||||||||||

This book is dedicated to my best
friend
and the love of my life, Jean.

Thank you for all of your support
and belief in me and in this project.

Introduction

||||||||||||||||||||||||||||||||||||||||||||||||||||||||||||||||||||||||||||||||||

Why Do We Need Another Weight-Loss Book?

The United States is experiencing an obesity epidemic. One aspect of this epidemic is an alarming increase in the incidence of type 2 diabetes mellitus. For the first time in U.S. history, this disease, which used to be called "adult-onset diabetes," is occurring in children and teens. Another sign of the times is the fact that ambulance companies, hospitals, makers of children's car seats, and even casket manufacturers have been forced to supersize their equipment and products to accommodate larger American bodies. According to the Centers for Disease Control and Prevention (CDC), more than 71 percent of American men weigh too much, along with 61 percent of women and 33 percent of children. Obesity is fast approaching tobacco as the number one cause of preventable death in the United States. The price tag to taxpayers, according to the CDC, is $117 billion a year. Moreover, Americans are spending a whopping $33 billion a year in their often futile attempts to become thinner.

It is time for a revolutionary approach to weight loss! Weight-loss books and diet franchises are a standard part of our culture, but they have had little impact on the obesity epidemic. The lack of success of previous books on this subject stems from three factors: First, authors, and experts in general, are asking the wrong question about obesity; second, the old paradigms accepted as gospel regarding weight management revolve around calorie-counting and exchange lists, concepts that do not work for 60 to 75 percent of overweight individuals; and finally, many authors are not sufficiently experienced

1

or skilled in the science of weight management (bariatrics) and have little data and no long-term follow-up program that might support their theories.

ııl Asking the Wrong Question

Advocates of The Zone, Ornish, Atkins, and South Beach diets, among others, approach the obesity problem with the wrong question in mind. They all ask: What is the one diet that Americans should follow for optimal weight loss? Based on the new understanding of genomics and nutrigenomics, medical concepts I will explain in this book, we now realize there never will be a single "one-size-fits-all" diet. Taking into consideration the genetic, ethnic, and lifestyle diversity of our American culture, this book demonstrates the key to successful weight management is tailoring a multifaceted nutrition, diet, and lifestyle program to meet the individual's unique biochemistry and metabolic needs. We never have had and never will find one diet or food plan that succeeds for everyone.

For example, an overweight reader might read an Atkins-type book and try the high-protein, low-carbohydrate diet advocated in that literature. There are several metabolic issues highlighted in my book that explain why a significant number of readers do not respond to an Atkins intervention. Examples include having a food hypersensitivity/allergy to eggs and milk or having a T4-T3 conversion problem in their thyroid pathway. Our book's questionnaires and clearly written chapters on these commonly overlooked forms of "switched metabolism" should alert readers to understand their failures and redirect their sights on more fruitful alternatives. Perhaps a reader has attempted the South Beach Diet and is frustrated that this approach failed to provide much-desired success. Hypothetically, our book could help them to understand that they could have a hormonal imbalance called estrogen dominance or perhaps a case of polycystic ovary syndrome (PCOS) that needs to be addressed; reading our book will help them to understand why the South Beach Diet alone could not succeed. Another reader may have tried Ann Louise Gittleman's Fat Flush Plan and was unable to achieve a meaningful response. Our book will point out that critical undiagnosed problems like leaky gut syndrome or unappreciated side effects from a prescribed medication were compromising weight-loss metabolism. Although Weight Watcher's and Jenny Craig have helped many people, millions have not responded. This book will help explain why these relatively high-glycemic-index diets are ineffective for insulin resistance or its preliminary metabolic impairment called *carbohydrate sensitivity*. Many of these nonresponders may be unaware of how chronic high stress levels produce adrenal gland overproduction of stress hormones that can cause weight-loss resistance.

ıl Let's Get Out of the Box

Americans have long been told, depending on the book and the system that is featured, that their obesity problem could easily be solved if they could only count. That is, by counting the number of calories, fat grams, protein grams, or carbohydrates you ingest, you can attain a healthy and normal weight. This book explains why these approaches have limited applicability and may be effective in only one-fourth to one-third of our obese population.

Instead, I have learned that five common metabolic issues plague 60 to 75 percent of obese Americans. Some people are affected by more than one of these metabolic compromises. Their ability to store fat instead of burning it, due to their biochemical individuality, does not conform to simple calorie counting, dietary exchange lists, or other conventional methods.

It is time for a revolution in the weight-loss industry! It is time to get out of the box and recognize that carbohydrate sensitivity, metabolic syndrome (a condition featuring too much insulin coupled with insulin resistance), hormonal imbalances, food hypersensitivities, and impaired liver detoxification are five common metabolic issues that are typically overlooked. This book explains how we can diagnose and successfully treat all of these common contributors to obesity.

ıl Who Am I to Say So?

Another reason I decided it was time for me to write *The Ultimate Metabolism Diet* is that I am a dedicated weight-loss specialist (bariatrician). I have dealt with this problem with great passion and energy for many years. I have seen hundreds of seriously overweight patients year after year since the early 1980s and have documented numerous cases that support my therapeutic paradigm; many cases with long-term follow-up are part of my database. My careful scrutiny of other well-known, best-selling weight-loss books, on the other hand, reveals the authors have had surprisingly little professional contact with overweight patients. Frequently these authors are cardiologists, researchers, pathologists, or exercise physiologists who have general knowledge and information about obesity and who tend to document their claims with generalized anecdotes and scant data. The standard popular weight-loss book presents no long-term follow-up, which is the true test of any successful weight-management theory. This book proposes to set a new standard and raise the bar with careful documentation, significant data, and long-term follow-up.

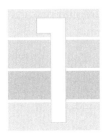

What Is
Switched Metabolism?

ιΙ Glossary of Medical Terms Used in Chapter 1

bariatric medicine: The medical specialty that deals with the diagnosis and treatment of obesity and related medical and nutritional problems.

carbohydrate sensitivity: A tendency for some people to react to simple carbohydrates such as processed white bread, sugar, white potatoes, or refined grain cereals with an exaggerated release of sugar into the bloodstream after eating; this in turns provokes the body to release extra insulin to help the body to process the blood sugar.

endocrine glands: Glands in the body that secrete hormonal substances into the bloodstream that can influence multiple areas of body functioning; examples are the thyroid and adrenal glands.

food hypersensitivity: An abnormal reaction of the immune system to certain trigger foods in the diet. This reaction involves excessive release of antibodies from the immune system that are usually provoked by microbes or pollens. These reactions can cause the release of toxins that can cause symptoms such headaches, skin rash, aches and pains, congestion, stomach problems, fluid retention and weight gain.

functional medicine: A new field of medicine that employs nutrition and lifestyle assessment and interventions to improve physiological, physical, and emotional/cognitive function.

genomics: The study of our genome, the sum of our 46 chromosomes, and the genes on these chromosomes; this gives information on how our DNA can be expressed in different ways to affect our body and health.

glycemic index: Measures the speed at which the body digests food, primarily carbohydrates, and converts it to blood sugar (glucose); the faster the food breaks down, the higher its rating on the index.

liver detoxification: The process by which the liver protects us from toxins in the environment and in our diet that circulate throughout our bloodstream. These toxins come from our food, water, and air; on a more subtle level, these toxins can originate from toxins manufactured in our bodies, microbes, and prescription drugs.

metabolic syndrome: A common cause of obesity seen in the apple-shaped body type; too much insulin in the body, which is not effective because of insulin resistance, characterizes it; these overweight people often have borderline blood sugar, high blood pressure, high triglycerides and low HDL, and are prediabetic.

metabolism: The process by which food substances are handled in the body. In this book, metabolism particularly refers to the body's ability to efficiently break down food for energy (efficient metabolism) and other necessary bodily processes versus its tendency to store the calories from food (sluggish or slow metabolism).

nutriceuticals: Natural supplements developed to have specific physiological and/or pharmacological effects to help the body to achieve health.

nutrigenomics: The study of how different foods may interact with specific genes to modify the risk of common, chronic diseases like diabetes and obesity.

switched metabolism: An impaired metabolism in which the person's body is preferentially storing calories consumed in the diet as fat for that proverbial "rainy day."

xenobiotics: Chemical substances that are foreign, and usually harmful, to the organism (e.g., PCPs).

■||||||||||||||||||||||||■

This book is for the frustrated, misunderstood, and often overmedicated overweight or obese person who has failed countless times to control his or her weight. A sacred tenet of popular weight-loss schemes for years has been that obesity could be solved if a person would, in a more careful or disciplined way, consume fewer calories and burn more calories. And depending on one's genetic makeup, I agree that the formula of "weight control = calories in – calories out" can work. Unfortunately, millions of Americans do not have this genetic makeup. They have tried, usually with great futility, every version of calorie-counting manipulation, consulting registered dietitians, medical doctors, commercial weight-loss franchises, and self-help books. Calorie counting for people with a *switched metabolism* has not achieved positive results. Simple math tells us these individuals are consuming far fewer calories than are assumed to be necessary to support their present body weight. Nevertheless, they do not lose weight at these lowered caloric levels and often continue to steadily gain weight.

> There are millions of Americans who do not have the genetic makeup to be successful with calorie counting.

Calorie counting has failed millions of Americans who are getting heavier and unhealthier. They take more medications and become part of our diabetes, hypertension, and heart disease epidemic statistics. Overweight or obese people with switched metabolism are trapped in a vicious cycle of storing fat for that "rainy day" that never comes. They have unique biochemical, metabolic, and genetic issues that cause their bodies to store fat instead of burning it. This book will help you to identify the five metabolic groups that cause switched metabolism. You will be able to identify which group or groups are causing your own overweight set point. Then you will learn, in practical terms, how to tailor a program to address your particular metabolic issues and to achieve outstanding results.

> Switched metabolism traps overweight people in a vicious cycle of storing fat instead of burning it.

Many years of clinical practice and research have helped us develop screening questionnaires that can help you categorize yourself as belonging to one or more of five metabolically impaired groups who suffer from switched metabolism. These include: (1) *carbohydrate sensitivity*; (2) *metabolic syndrome* (also known as insulin resistance syndrome and syndrome X); (3) *functional hormonal imbalances*; (4) *food hypersensitivities*; and (5) *impaired liver detoxification* (usually associated with a chronic illness). In each of these conditions, you will learn that it is the type of calories—not just the total number of calories—that is critical in determining whether your body stores or burns fat.

Five Metabolic Groups That Cause Switched Metabolism

1. carbohydrate sensitivity
2. metabolic syndrome
3. functional endocrine abnormalities
4. food hypersensitivities
5. impaired liver detoxification

Our program is based on cutting-edge developments and innovations in the fields of biochemistry, genetics, and nutrition that will be discussed in detail later in the book. These advances include the following developments:

- The functional medicine approach and philosophy facilitates thinking about new approaches to the problem of obesity.

- New biochemical understanding states how the type of calories you eat, not just the total number of calories consumed, can be critical to whether you store or burn fat.

- New strategies are under development to balance thyroid, adrenal, and sex hormones.

- Elucidation of metabolic syndrome, a problem that involves "apple" or upper-body obesity, abnormal insulin, and blood sugar imbalance, often including elevated blood pressure, elevated triglycerides, and low HDL cholesterol. (Metabolic syndrome, which is often a precursor to diabetes mellitus type 2, is said to affect one out of every four to five American adults.)

- Pioneering work is occurring in the field of allergy and immunology, showing the effect of food hypersensitivities on weight-loss metabolism.

- There is increased understanding of the role of liver detoxification in chronic illness, helping to explain why many people gain significant weight after developing a chronic illness, such as chronic fatigue syndrome (CFS) and fibromyalgia (FM).

- Numerous breakthroughs are occurring in the development of nutriceutical products, which are natural supplements developed to correct abnormal physiology. We are using several of these new products that have been developed to address obesity and metabolic problems. Our patients have received great benefits from these new products, without experiencing any negative side effects from medications.

Pioneered by Dr. Jeffrey Bland and his colleagues, the functional medicine approach to obesity and other medical problems has inspired a revolutionary approach that has helped hundreds of patients in my medical practice. It is a new field of medicine that employs nutrition and lifestyle assessment and intervention to improve physiological, emotional/cognitive, and physical function.

ııl Dynamics of Functional Medicine

In functional medicine, we feel the key to understanding and treating the obesity epidemic is to think outside the box by adopting a new focus. The individual—not the disease—is the target of treatment. The focus, instead, is on understanding the breakdown of mechanisms that help one maintain a healthy body weight.

Sidney Baker, MD, author of *Detoxification and Healing: The Key to Optimal Health*, explains: "People do not get sick from diseases, but rather diseases reflect a disruption in the dynamic balance between themselves and their environment." Fundamental to functional medicine is an awareness of the web-like interactions among all systems in the body. These web-like connections of physiological factors explain that a patient has a dynamic balance that can be upset by a number of external factors such as allergens, xenobiotics, drugs, endotoxins, diet, and emotional stress. Functional medicine emphasizes that lifestyle translates into quantifiable effects on health and disease through the energetics of our biochemistry and genetics. In contrast to traditional medical, functional medicine emphasizes health as a positive vitality, not merely the absence of disease.

From the functional medicine perspective, patient care recognizes that each person has a unique biochemical and genetic structure. From mapping the genome, researchers discovered that there are at least 100 obesity genes that can combine to express themselves in myriad ways, as well as 300 diabetic genes. Thus, the functional medicine position is that science never will be able to adopt a cookie-cutter approach to weight management or a one-size-fits-all paradigm. Simply stated, functional medicine maintains there will never be just one diet, one pill, or one natural supplement that will address the concerns of all overweight persons. Each overweight person's biochemical individuality must be acknowledged and addressed.

Glycemic index, genomics, and nutrigenomics are terms I will use repeatedly in the book. You may not be familiar with these terms. The *glycemic index* (GI) measures the speed at which you digest food and convert it to glucose (blood sugar), your body's energy source. The faster the food breaks down, the higher its rating on the index. The index sets glucose at 100 and scores all foods against that number. Low-glycemic-index foods are slower to digest, so you feel satiated longer. Low-glycemic-index foods also help keep insulin levels low, which inhibits the formation of fat and assists in the conversion of fat back into energy.

Genomics is the study of the genome—the sum of our 46 chromosomes and the genes on these chromosomes—and how our DNA can be expressed in different ways to affect our physiologic function and anatomical expression. The study of genomics has yielded amazing knowledge, such as the fact that there are more than 100 obesity genes that can combine and interact in a myriad of ways to express many different phenotypes (outer physical expressions) of obesity.

Nutrigenomics is the study of how different foods can interact with specific genes to modify the risk of common chronic diseases such as type 2 diabetes, obesity, heart disease, stroke, and certain cancers. Nutrigenomics also seeks to identify the biologically active molecules in the diet that affect health by altering the expression of genes. The premise underlying nutrigenomics is that the influence of diet on health is related to an individual's genetic makeup. Scientists now state unequivocally that "genes in and of themselves do not create disease. Only when they are plunged into a harmful environment unique to the individual do they create the outcome of disease."[1] Nutrigenomics is based on the premise that nutrients serve as dietary signals that modify gene expression, protein synthesis, and metabolic function.

ıI Dilemma of the Pima Indians

A clear example of the application of genomics and nutrigenomics is the dilemma of the Pima Indians, a dramatic case of the ways environment and lifestyle influence gene expression and subsequent cellular function. The branch of the Pima tribe centered in Arizona has extreme problems with obesity and diabetes, while the Pima Indians in Mexico have virtually no such medical problems. DNA analysis has proven the two groups are indeed genetically identical. The difference clearly can be explained in their different lifestyles, which subsequently put their genes into radically different environments that lead to differing clinical expression. The Pima in Mexico live as their ancestors have for hundreds of years, eating native desert plants and wild game, and scratching out a subsistence living from the soil, which requires a high level of physical activity. They have no fast foods, vending machines, or modern supermarkets. As the Arizona Pima abandoned their ancestral diets in favor of a "modern" diet high in fat, sugar, and processed foods, however, their incidence of diabetes and obesity rapidly escalated. Interestingly, prior to 1940, the Arizona Pima lived more traditionally and suffered no more obesity and diabetes than other Americans. Clearly, the same set of genes and genetic tendencies can express obesity tendencies differently depending on the environment in which we place them.

ıI The "Last-Resort" Doctor

As a board-certified specialist in the fields of bariatrics and family practice, I have treated hundreds of overweight patients, integrating the new nutritional, genomic, and biochemical developments that are the core of the functional medicine philosophy. In terms of weight management, I have become a "last-resort doctor." That is, desperately overweight people come to see me as the "last resort." Each person I see with a diagnosis of obesity is in reality an expression of his or her unique biochemical individuality and genomics. Identifying and understanding the underlying mechanisms for each case inevitably leads to different strategies for varying clinical presentations that are much more likely to be successful. One of the ways I will help you understand this integration will be through the use of actual clinical case studies. I believe these case studies will not only be interesting and inspiring, but they will also explain and document how this revolutionary system works.

Before I present the first story of one of my patients, I would like to define some terms you will see in these patient stories. Upper-body, abdominal, or "apple" obesity is defined by a waist circumference of greater than 35 inches in females and 40 inches in males. This parameter correlates highly with insulin resistance and metabolic syndrome. Individuals with "apple" obesity have a much higher incidence of heart disease, diabetes, and certain cancers than others of the same height and weight and more a "pear" distribution of body fat. An acceptable blood pressure is < 130/90, a more optimal one is under 120/80. A fasting blood sugar level lower than 100 is desirable, 100–126 is borderline for diabetes, and above 126 indicates the patient is diabetic. Random blood sugar tests or two-hour blood sugar tests (usually taken after drinking 75 grams of glucola in the lab) should be under 200, with < 160 as more optimal. Fasting insulin levels should ideally be 8 or less, and two-hour insulin levels should be under 50. Acceptable total cholesterol should be less than 200, with optimal being 160–180. HDL, the good cholesterol fraction, should be above 50 for females and 40 for males, and the higher the better. LDL, the bad or clogging cholesterol fraction, should be below 130 and optimally below 100. Triglycerides, a different kind of fat more related to carbohydrate and sugar intake, should be under 150, with under 100 being optimal. CRP-hs (also called C-reactive protein) is a measure of inflammation in the coronary arteries and should be under 3.0, with an optimal level of less than 1.0. Homocysteine is a coronary risk factor related to inherited abnormal metabolism of the amino acid methionine. It should be under 8. A triglyceride/HDL ratio is a good predictor of insulin resistance in a patient. Any ratio of 4 or higher is highly suspect.

Optimal Tests and Measurement Values

Waist circumference	Males: under 40 inches	Females: under 36 inches
Blood pressure	Acceptable: 130/90	Optimal: 120/80
Fasting blood sugar (mg/dL)	Optimal: under 100	Borderline: 100–126
Two-hour blood sugar (mg/dL)	Acceptable: under 200	Optimal: under 160
Fasting insulin	Optimal: under 8	
Two-hour insulin	Optimal: under 50	
Cholesterol	Acceptable: 200	Optimal: 160–180
HDL (mg/dL)	Optimal (males) 40+	Optimal (females): 50+,
LDL (mg/dL)	Acceptable: 100–130	Optimal: under 100
Triglycerides (mg/dL)	Acceptable: under 150	Optimal: under 100
CRP-hs	Acceptable: under 3.0	Optimal: under 1.0
Homocysteine	Optimal: under 8	
Triglyceride/HDL ratio	Optimal: under 4.0	

Ernie's Story

Losing Weight to Gain a New Life

Ernie is a 45-year-old male who came to our office with severe obesity that was resistant to vigorous weight-loss efforts (otherwise known as refractory obesity). He had the upper body "apple" distribution, which is associated with severe cravings for sugars and starches.

He had been unsuccessful in losing weight on popular high-protein, low-carbohydrate diets. He also had numerous medical problems, including a heart condition called atrial fibrillation that required a pacemaker. In addition to high blood pressure, Ernie also had severe osteoarthritis and abnormal liver function tests. Ernie was on multiple prescriptions for his blood pressure, heart, blood, and thyroid. He spent most of his day resting or in bed. He had not been able to work for several years due to his failing health.

Ernie's Initial Evaluation

Height: 5 feet, 10 inches

Weight: 384.5 pounds

Blood pressure: 132/91 (normal limit (nl):130/80)

Ernie's cholesterol, triglycerides, and LDL cholesterol levels were all normal, but his HDL was 28, which is far below the minimal desirable level of 50.

Triglyceride/HDL ratio: 5.3 (nl: 4.0)

The results of laboratory tests showed that Ernie had extremely high insulin levels:

Fasting insulin: 93.5 (nl: 8)

Two-hour insulin: 433.2 (nl: 25)

The results of the blood sugar tests showed that Ernie was in the borderline diabetic range:

Fasting blood sugar: 123 (nl: 100)

Two-hour blood sugar: 186 (nl: 160)

His TSH (a test of the activity of the thyroid) was mildly elevated, indicating he was on too low a dose of thyroid medication.

TSH: 6.10 (nl: 4.50)

Initial Assessment

Our initial assessment focused on Ernie's having metabolic syndrome, borderline diabetes mellitus, borderline thyroid status, and severe refractory obesity.

Recommendations

We then recommended that Ernie begin taking the following steps:

1. Begin a low-glycemic-index 1,600–1,800 calorie diet with six meals daily.
2. Begin a specially configured soy-based protein formula with slow-release starch (high-amylose starch), which causes a low blood sugar and insulin response, two scoops given twice daily.
3. Drink 64–80 ounces of water daily.
4. Increase thyroid medication to a dose of L-thyroxin 225 mcg daily.
5. Start nutritional supplementation for support of blood sugar and insulin, including chromium 200 mcg daily, vanadyl sulfate

7.5 mg daily, magnesium malate 250 mg twice daily, and conjugated linoleic acid (CLA) 1 gram daily.

6. Begin walking 4 minutes four or five times daily inside the house.
7. Keep careful daily records of food intake, symptoms, and activity.
8. Return to our office regularly for visits for monitoring, patient education, and support.
9. Conduct sleep studies to see if patient has obstructive sleep apnea.

6-Week Follow-Up

Ernie's weight is 372 pounds, showing a loss of 12.6 pounds. His blood pressure is 120/80. A sleep study shows a severe case of apnea. The home monitoring of fasting blood sugar is consistently 80–120.

Plan: Add a fiber product containing psyllium and 7.5 grams of guar gum, one scoop daily; implement CPAP machine for sleep apnea per pulmonologist's instructions.

12-Week Follow-Up

Ernie's weight is 355 pounds. He lost an additional 17 pounds for a total of 29.6 pounds, so far. His fasting blood sugar is 77, his fasting insulin is 17, and his TSH is 3.81. He is now able to perform some light household tasks.

Plan: Continue the same program.

28-Week Follow-Up

Ernie's weight is 293.6 pounds (total loss of 91 pounds); his blood pressure is 104/72. Ernie continues to feel stronger and is now seldom napping during the day.

One-Year Follow-Up

Ernie's weight is 240 pounds (total loss of 135 pounds). Ernie has resumed some activities, including motorcycle riding and taking a few adult education classes.

Plan: Continue same program.

Two-Year Follow-Up

Because his symptoms of lethargy and brain fog have greatly improved, Ernie is taking 12 credit hours at the community college and receiving excellent grades.

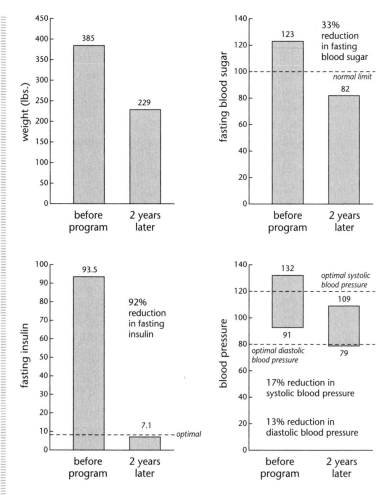

FIGURES 1.1 THROUGH 1.4. Ernie's reduction in weight, blood sugar, insulin, and blood pressure

Summary

	INITIAL	FINAL
Weight	384.5 pounds	229.4 pounds
Blood pressure	132/91	109/79
Fasting blood sugar	231	82
Fasting insulin	93.5	7.1

Comments

This is a remarkable tribute to one man's patience, persistence, and willingness to try a new approach. After several physicians told Ernie he was a "hopeless case," he truly reinvented himself in a number of ways. His weight loss of 154.8 pounds, averaging a little over two pounds a week for two years, is amazing. He has lowered his blood pressure 23 points, improved his blood sugar 41 points, and normalized one of the highest insulin levels we have seen in our facility. His initial TSH thyroid lab test showed that even on medication, his thyroid function was sluggish. It is noteworthy that with an adjustment in medication, his thyroid status has normalized from a TSH of 6.10 to 3.81.

Key Idea

Ernie is a very large individual, who lost over 150 pounds. It is inspiring to know that there is hope for such difficult and extreme cases of obesity. What you need to know is that *the principles explained in this book will work for anyone, whether they need to lose 10 or 50 or 100 pounds!*

ııl The Obesity Crisis Is an Opportunity

Our country is in a health-care crisis regarding obesity. More than 61 percent of adults are overweight, and 27 percent of them—50 million people—are obese according to the U.S. Surgeon General's report. For the first time, obesity has surpassed smoking as the leading cause of preventable death in our country. Sadly, 400,000 people have died over the past year due the ravages of obesity, almost one person every 75 seconds! It has been well documented that obesity is an independent major risk factor for heart disease and that it is associated with increased risk for stroke, diabetes, hypertension, elevated cholesterol and triglycerides, blood clots and pulmonary emboli, gall bladder disease, and osteoarthritis. In the past few years, additional research has clarified that obesity is also highly associated with cancer, especially cancer associated with the colon, prostate, and the female organs. Moreover, obesity is implicated in polycystic ovary syndrome, urinary incontinence, and complications of pregnancy. Amazingly, obesity has recently surpassed alcohol as the leading cause of liver disease, as it is often associated with a fatty liver condition called steatosis. Obesity is a leading cause of the common sleep disorder called obstructive sleep apnea, and it is associated with increased rates of depression.

New research has shown that obesity is an inflammatory state, with fat cells stimulating the release of cytokines (chemicals that cause aching muscles and joints and coronary artery inflammation), thereby accelerating arteriosclerosis. This effect is evidenced by the correlation of elevated CRP-hs, which is a marker for coronary artery inflammation that is more prevalent in overweight and obese individuals. A recent study even shows that obesity is associated with hormonal changes that can adversely affect male erectile function.

Medical Conditions Related to Obesity

- heart disease
- gallbladder disease
- stroke
- osteoarthritis
- diabetes
- certain cancers
- hypertension
- polycystic ovary syndrome
- abnormal cholesterol
- abnormal triglycerides
- blood clots
- urinary incontinence
- fatty liver (steatosis)
- complication of pregnancy
- sleep apnea
- depression
- fatigue
- erectile dysfunction

The amount obesity costs our society is staggering. In 2003 the United States spent more than $99 billion in the treatment of obesity and its related conditions. An informal study in our office indicated the typical obese adult was taking prescriptions for obesity-related problems totaling a retail value of $418 per month, which amounts to over $5,000 a year! The cost in human suffering due to impaired self-esteem and relationship issues, in addition to professional and social discrimination, is incalculable.

Obviously, it is time for new ideas and new approaches. The definition of insanity has been said to be the repetition of the same behavior over and over while expecting different results. I invite you to continue reading the subsequent chapters to find out how you, and many others in our country with serious obesity-related problems, can now begin to move forward. You can avoid fitting this definition of insanity by changing your procedure!

ıl Screening Questionnaires Are the Key

The screening questionnaires below, which are repeated at the beginnings of Chapters 3 through 7, are the key to the reader getting the most from this book. By completing these questionnaires and comparing your score to the answer key, you will identify the areas of switched metabolism that need to be addressed. Some readers may clearly need help in only one of the areas of metabolic impairment, while others may have two or three areas of compromised metabolism.

ıl Functional Medicine Weight Management Screening Questionnaire

Part I: Carbohydrate Sensitivity
Circle the number of any statement that applies to you.

1. I eat out 10 or more times in a week.

2. I consume 14 or more alcoholic drinks in a week.

3. I seldom eat more than two servings (combined) of fruits and vegetables daily.

4. I consume more than 20 ounces of soft drink daily.

5. I seldom exercise 60 minutes or more in a week.

6. I consume refined sugar/carbohydrates at least several times daily.

7. I frequently eat between meals.

8. I consume foods such as hamburgers, hot dogs, pizza, fried chicken, fries, or chips almost every day.

9. I have a problem with stress eating or compulsive eating.

Answer Key: If you have circled four or more statements, your lifestyle and genetics have probably combined to create carbohydrate sensitivity as a major factor in perpetuating your weight problem and keeping you from succeeding in a weight-loss program. It is imperative that as part of your program you carefully evaluate and implement the ideas presented in Chapter 3.

Part II: Metabolic Syndrome
Circle the number of any statement that applies to you.

1. My family history is positive for diabetes mellitus.
2. My medical history is positive for high triglycerides.
3. My medical history is positive for infertility, unwanted facial hair, or ovarian cysts.
4. I frequently crave sugar and/or carbohydrates.
5. I experience erratic energy and/or mood swings that can be affected by eating.
6. I gain weight in the upper body or have an "apple" body shape.
7. I have experienced gestational diabetes and/or have delivered a baby who weighed more than 9 pounds.
8. My medical history is positive for borderline or confirmed high blood pressure.
9. My medical history is positive for gout and/or elevated uric acid.
10. My medical history is positive for borderline blood sugar readings.
11. My ethnic roots are non-European.
12. I have multiple tiny moles or "skin tags" on my upper body and neck.

Answer Key: If you circled five or more statements, your lifestyle and genomics have probably combined to create metabolic syndrome as a major factor in perpetuating your weight problem and keeping you from success in a weight-loss program. It is imperative that as part of your program you carefully evaluate and implement the ideas presented in Chapter 4.

Part III: Hormonal Imbalances
Circle the number of any statement that applies to you.

A. For Men and Women

1. My family history is positive for thyroid problems.
2. I frequently feel cold when others are comfortable.
3. My face and body are often puffy or swollen.

4. I am very sluggish in the morning and have difficulty in getting up.

5. My hair appears to be unhealthy or is falling out.

6. My skin has become overly dry.

7. My nails are brittle.

8. I have a history of high cholesterol.

9. I am taking Synthroid or another thyroid replacement.

10. I have significant issues with decreased libido.

11. My weight gain has coincided with very high stress.

12. I have gained weight in my upper back below the neck level.

B. *For Women Only*

1. I experience food cravings and weight gain with PMS.

2. My weight gain has been associated with perimenopause or menopause.

3. My weight gain has been associated with taking hormone replacement therapy or the birth control pill.

4. I have abnormal menstrual cycles.

5. I have had difficulty getting pregnant.

6. I have had ovarian cysts, documented either by ultrasound and/or laparoscopy.

7. My menstrual cycles usually are very uncomfortable/painful.

8. Unwanted facial hair has become a problem.

9. I have had thinning of the hair on the top of my head.

10. I have had a tendency to have acne and/or seborrhea (dandruff).

11. I have continued to gain weight even though I have tried to reduce.

12. I tend to carry my body fat in the "apple" distribution.

13. I have skin tags around my neck and upper body.

14. I have been told my blood sugar is abnormal or borderline.

15. I have had to take birth control pills or have had surgery for gynecological symptoms.

Answer Key: If you have circled five or more statements in part A, your lifestyle and genomics have probably combined to create hormonal abnormalities as a major factor in perpetuating your weight problem and keeping you from success in a weight-loss program. If you have circled two or more statements from questions 1–3 in part B, it is likely that you have estrogen dominance, a type of hormonal imbalance that contributes to switched metabolism. If you have circled five or more statements from questions 4–15 in part B, you likely have polycystic ovary syndrome (PCOS). Carefully evaluate the ideas presented in Chapter 5.

Part IV: Food Hypersensitivity

Circle the numbers of any statements that apply to you.

1. As an infant or small child I had problems with colic, allergies, or recurrent respiratory infections.
2. I have a past or current medical history of asthma.
3. I have a past or current medical history of chronic nasal or sinus problems.
4. I have a past or current medical history of hives or eczema.
5. I have a past or current medical history of irritable bowel syndrome.
6. I have a past or current medical history of excessive headaches.
7. I have a past or current medical history of musculoskeletal aches and pains.
8. I eat wheat or milk-based foods several times a day.

Answer Key: If you have circled three items, it is possible that food hypersensitivities are contributing to your weight problem. If you have circled four or more items, it is likely you have significant food hypersensitivities that are contributing to your weight problem and switched metabolism. Carefully evaluate the ideas presented in Chapter 6.

Part V: Liver Detoxification/Weight Gain with Chronic Illness

Circle the number of any statement that applies to you.

1. I started gaining weight after I contracted a chronic illness.

2. I have a chronic illness (e.g., chronic fatigue syndrome, fibromyalgia, rheumatoid arthritis).
3. I frequently feel exhausted.
4. I frequently feel sick all over, like having the flu or mono.
5. I am very sensitive to medications.
6. I am very sensitive to smoke, chemicals, or fumes in the environment.
7. I am taking or have in the past taken a lot of prednisone, nonsteroidal anti-inflammatory drugs (NSAIDS, such as Motrin, Advil, ibuprofen), antibiotics, antidepressants, or other medications.
8. My illness causes me to be quite sedentary.
9. I have had frequent yeast infections (including thrush).

Answer Key: If you have circled four items, it is possible that impaired liver detoxification is contributing to your weight problem; if you have circled five or more items, it is likely that significant issues with impaired liver detoxification are contributing to your weight problem and switched metabolism. Carefully evaluate the ideas presented in Chapter 7.

ιII How to Proceed after Completing the Questionnaires

If you score positively on the screening questionnaires for both carbohydrate sensitivity and metabolic syndrome, you should prioritize the program designed for metabolic syndrome. Metabolic syndrome is more medically serious and represents advanced progression of metabolic impairment that usually begins after many years of carbohydrate sensitivity. In this case, you are particularly encouraged to read about carbohydrate sensitivity in Chapter 3. There is a lot of very helpful information, as well as inspiring patient stories, in each chapter. Regardless of your questionnaire score, read each chapter so you do not miss out on this information. In addition, most readers can learn something practical and useful from Chapter 8, which deals with emotional eating.

ııl What If I Have Multiple Areas of Switched Metabolism?

If you have a positive questionnaire response to multiple areas of switched metabolism, work on them sequentially in the order they are presented in the book: carbohydrate sensitivity (Chapter 3), metabolic syndrome (Chapter 4), hormonal imbalances (Chapter 5), food hypersensitivities (Chapter 6), and impaired liver detoxification (Chapter 7). For example, if you have issues with carbohydrate sensitivity and/or metabolic syndrome plus hormonal imbalances and food hypersensitivities, work on metabolic syndrome or carbohydrate sensitivity for 60 days, then add the hormonal imbalance protocols for 60 days, followed by the food hypersensitivity protocols for 60 days. Another example of multiple areas of switched metabolism would be an individual needing to improve hormonal imbalances, food hypersensitivities, and liver detoxification. The recommended sequential approach would be 60 days on hormonal imbalances, followed by 60 days on food hypersensitivities, followed by 60 days on liver detoxification. **The rule of thumb is: Work on one area of switched metabolism for 60 days before adding the next area of metabolic need for 60 days.**

Unless you have a professional who can skillfully help you combine multiple approaches, it is too overwhelming to work on everything at once. If you need outside assistance, physicians from the American Society of Bariatric Physicians (www.asbp.org) and the Institute of Functional Medicine (www.fxmed.com) can help you integrate these approaches, providing wisdom and understanding.

Ready...Set...Go!

ıl Glossary of Medical Terms Used in Chapter 2

aldosterone: A hormone secreted by the adrenal gland that can affect sodium and fluid retention.

hyperlipidemia: Excess fats (or lipids) in the bloodstream such as cholesterol and triglycerides.

triglycerides: A type of fat circulating in the bloodstream that is derived from fatty acids made by the liver in response to the intake of blood sugar. These can, in some cases, become excessive and contribute to blockages in the blood vessels.

ıl Weight Loss and Hiking the Grand Canyon

What does hiking the Grand Canyon successfully have in common with your successful weight-loss program? Experienced hikers know that to be successful in hiking a challenging trail in the Grand Canyon, it is imperative to be prepared mentally, emotionally, and physically. Planning is paramount. You must know the trail, its elevation changes, likely weather patterns, and the typical time and effort required to safely navigate the trail. Moreover, if you want to hike the Grand Canyon safely and successfully, you need to understand how to train for the experience, know the water and food requirements, and be clear on what clothing and footwear will likely contribute to success. I have seen enthusiastic, well-intentioned hikers on the trails in the Grand Canyon in sandals with no socks, carrying only a small thermos of orange juice for hydration, and wearing black clothing on a hot summer day. Because of their lack of understanding of the basic necessities of success, these unfortunate people did not finish the hike and they often had to be rescued by helicopter.

ııl Good Preparation Is Your Key to Success

Similarly, to succeed on the rocky road to weight management success, it is important to know what basic prerequisites are required for a successful journey. For your program to work, you must:

1. Have the commitment to do whatever it takes to succeed.
2. Implement the daily general principles of maintaining a successful program.
3. Understand your personal triggers for inappropriate eating.
4. Keep careful, daily lifestyle records.
5. Understand how the "Five Ps" will teach you a winning attitude.
6. Embrace the power of walking regularly.
7. Remember to drink water.

ıl 1. Commitment to Your Program Leads to Success

Sign Your Personal Weight-Loss Contract

To make certain this will be the final, permanently successful program to control your weight, it is crucial for you to consider carefully your commitment and motivation. Obviously, without commitment and positive motivation, no program can succeed. Begin by reading and signing your personal weight-loss contract. This contract symbolically affirms your sincere desire to implement the ideas in this book and documents your pledge to change your life.

Post your contract in a prominent spot, such as on your bathroom mirror or refrigerator, where you can read it regularly. Carry a copy with you.

Here is a sample of a weight-loss contract. Make your own contract that reflects your personal goals and motivations.

My Personal Weight-Loss Contract

My weight today is: _____

My goal weight in 4 weeks is: _____

My goal weight in 12 weeks is: _____

My goal weight in 6 months is: _____

My goal weight in 1 year is: _____

I, _____, sincerely dedicate myself to carry out the ideas in this book for the next year as closely as possible. I will earnestly strive to change my relationship with food and to make other recommended lifestyle changes. I will allow no excuses or conditions to prevent me from making a 100 percent effort.

Date: _____   Signed: _____

                         Witness: _____

List Ten Reasons Why You Want to Lose Weight
An invaluable exercise for our patients before they begin their weight-loss program is to list ten reasons why they want to lose weight. I advise each individual to give serious thought to this assignment. It is of the utmost importance that these ten reasons reflect your true goals and desires and are very personal to you. They should not be vague generalizations but rather should state specific outcomes. Do not worry about what would please others, but carefully consider what would please you.

These ten reasons will become your personal motivators. Each day, before you go to sleep, slowly read through your list. Some of these reasons may define conditions you want to leave behind forever. Other reasons will state in positive terms the experience you wish to have and a life condition you would like to achieve. Your mind will accept your suggestions for improvement.

In addition, copy your ten reasons onto a 3 × 5-inch index card and carry that card with you at all times. When you are confronted with a difficult situation or are filled with doubts and conflicts, read the entire list to give you a mental boost. Your ten reasons should be posted in several places where you will see them during the day, including the car, bathroom mirror, refrigerator, office desk, or wherever they might be helpful.

Why I Want to Lose Weight

1. _____

_____

2. _____

_____

3. _____

_____

4. _____

_____

5. _____

_____

6. _____

_____

7. _____

_____

8. _____

_____

9. _____

_____

10. _____

_____

ıl 2. General Principles of Success

Weigh yourself every four to seven days. Too frequent weighing can be confusing and play mind games with you. Over the long haul the scales will not lie. However, weighing daily or even more often can create an illusion. You can do everything "right," but due to momentary fluid shifts, hormone changes, or other factors, the scale may show only a slight or no improvement. This can lead to unnecessary discouragement or depression and the mistaken idea that your program is failing.

On the other hand, you could have a shaky adherence to successful principles but the scale may show improvement. Your subconscious mind is elated. The message is that a halfway performance is okay because "the scale shows I am getting away with it."

To avoid these pitfalls, remember to weigh yourself twice a week, but not on consecutive days. Always weigh yourself wearing similar clothes, at the same time of day, using the same scale. Also, remember there are a number of equally significant criteria besides the number on the scale that give you feedback. These include waist circumference, clothing size, improvement in physical and medical symptoms, body fat composition, laboratory data, and reduction or elimination of medications. If you are doing good things for your body and health consistently, the number on the scale will take care of itself.

Remove all danger foods from the home. Most obese people who come to our office agree there are particular foods they crave or tend to overeat. What are your danger foods? If you have these foods in the house, do yourself a favor and get rid of them. Throw them out or give them away. Over the course of the next year, do not purchase these foods or keep them in the house.

Plan your meals—write them out. When making significant lifestyle changes, it has been our experience that you will be less likely to shoot yourself in the foot if you streamline and structure the process of change. Keep things simple and structured by planning your meals and snacks for one week in advance. If you will be eating out, also design a written plan for that experience. Written shopping lists are very helpful. This is an excellent tool to use as you gain control of your new dietary lifestyle.

Drink a large glass of water prior to each meal. Not only is this a healthy habit in general, but it will also help fill your stomach and prevent overeating.

Eat your meals slowly. Many of us are in the bad habit of eating too quickly. Our stomach and brain are out of touch, and we do not know when true physiological hunger has been satisfied. Strive to make your meals last at least 20 minutes. If necessary, monitor the clock. Other useful techniques to slow down eating include chewing each bite 20 times and intentionally setting down your fork between bites. Actually getting up from the table for two or three minutes may also help. Remember to eat like a true gourmet!

Always leave some food. One of the strongest programmed messages that triggers compulsive overeating comes from our youth. We learned that to be a good child and win our parents' approval, we had to eat all the food on our plate. So, as adults, instead of stopping when we are full, we continue to stuff ourselves. To break this habit, always leave a bit of food on your plate.

Eat according to a simple, consistent routine. People with weight problems are often controlled by external cues in their environment. To establish inner control, develop the habit of eating at the same time and in the same place. Eat only from a plate, do not eat alone if you can avoid it, and do not eat while reading or listening to the radio or television. Instead, listen to your stomach.

Avoid the kitchen. We would not send a recovering alcoholic to the local bar to pick up some beer for us on a hot Saturday night. For similar reasons, we advise you to stay out of the kitchen except when it is absolutely necessary to prepare or clean up meals.

ıl 3. Triggers for Inappropriate Eating
Why Do You Want to Eat?

As you begin the exciting process of reinventing yourself in terms of what you eat and how you exercise, it is essential to evaluate and change your relationship with food. When I was struggling with my weight, someone asked me, "Why do you want to eat?" I laughed and replied, "I want to eat because the food is available and it tastes good!" Of course, I missed the point of the question. When we initiate eating behavior, what is going on? If we are truly biologically hungry, with symptoms of an empty stomach such as contractions, then eating is certainly appropriate. Make the best choice you can to eat healthfully and then move on. On the other hand, if you start asking yourself the key question, "Why do I want to eat?" throughout the day, you may frequently be surprised to learn you are initiating eating behavior that has nothing to do with true biological hunger.

> Cues that initiate eating behavior often have nothing to do with real hunger. Instead, they are likely to include stress, social pressures, boredom, fatigue, or the need for comfort.

Instead, the cues that initiate eating behavior often form a lengthy list, including stress, social situations (everybody else is eating), the feeling that it is time to eat, boredom, fatigue, needing comfort, associating eating with an activity like attending a ballgame, watching a movie, and so on.

To eat healthfully and in a way that ensures successful weight loss, you must master and understand your particular eating triggers. An effective technique is to post small signs or 3 × 5-inch index cards throughout your house, office, and car posing the question: "Why do I want to eat?" More important, make yourself answer this question every time before eating, with the goal of making eating a mindful activity, not just an automatic or unconscious one. If the answer to "Why do I want to eat?" is something other than true biological hunger, identify what you are experiencing and feeling, and ask a key follow-up question. Given what I am experiencing or feeling, what would be a more appropriate alternative behavior to eating?

Inappropriate Eating Behaviors

The following is an example of inappropriate eating behavior. A woman was anxious and depressed over the diagnosis of her brother's cancer. She and her brother had always been very close. When she came into the office, she had gained 10 pounds during the previous month, all of it related to inappropriate stress eating. She clearly identified that she wanted to eat because of stress. Obviously, the eating and weight gain were not helping either her ill brother or herself, so we listed a number of alternative constructive behaviors to substitute for her inappropriate eating behavior. These included preparing some meals and soup for her brother, taking him to some of his treatments, obtaining books and videos for him to help pass the time, and so on. And I facetiously commented that if I thought eating would truly help her brother with his cancer issues, I would be the first to pass out the chips and brownies to help speed his recovery! With perspective, we can all understand that eating has never helped solve a personal, family, or professional problem. Most of us have tried it and have experienced the futility.

In another example of inappropriate eating, a patient dealt with the problem by asking, "Why do I want to eat?" This gentleman was driving home from work and was stopped by the police for driving 35 m.p.h. in a 25 m.p.h. zone in the park near his home. He pleaded for a warning, but the officer informed him that warnings could only be given when the speed limit was exceeded by 9 miles or less. When he arrived home, he was in a bad mood. An hour after eating a normal evening meal, he was consuming leftovers. Another hour later, he was eating a banana. A little later, things really started to unravel when he began to eat a huge bowl of ice cream. Serendipitously, he looked up from his ice cream and was suddenly confronting his "Why do I want to eat?" sign on the refrigerator. Sheepishly, he recognized he had fallen into an old behav-

Why Do I Want to Eat?

1. If the answer to "Why do I want to eat?" is a reason other than true biological hunger, identify the trigger.

2. Then formulate an alternative behavior to inappropriate eating that responds to the trigger.

ior pattern and was eating, not due to hunger, but as an expression of anger and frustration. He used his new paradigm and asked himself what might be more appropriate behaviors to substitute for overeating. His options were to: go for a walk to release some of the anger and frustration; pay the fine, send the check in, and resolve the entire situation; set a date in court to plead his side of the case; make a date to attend traffic school to take the incident off his record; and buy a radar detector. We can debate the relative merits of these five alternatives, but they all make more sense than eating large amounts of food without even being hungry.

ıı 4. Keep Careful Daily Lifestyle Records

Keeping careful daily lifestyle records is a marvelous way to get immediate feedback about your relationship with food and other problem areas. Researchers find this type of self-monitoring correlates highly with success.

Record Keeping

Probably the most important lifestyle behavior we recommend is often the most underestimated, but we've found that daily record keeping correlates highly with success. This practice gives you a powerful feedback loop regarding such variables in your program as eating, exercise, and fluid intake. Your records will increase your awareness of eating and its effect on your weight. You are being asked to change your habits, and awareness is a key step in this process. The awareness you gain from record keeping has several benefits, including making better food selections, becoming more aware of what you eat, and increasing your control over eating by identifying feelings and activities related to food consumption. Depending on the person, we have seen excellent results from using small notebooks, individual record sheets, or word processing programs. Remember—a key to success is to immediately record food and liquid intake and exercise. Do not wait until the end of the day or the end of the week. Keep records as you go along.

The following is a sample of a form our patients have used called Weekly Record. Make your own copy to chart your weekly progress.

WEEKLY RECORD: **Week of:** _____   **Name:** _____

	Sunday	Monday	Tuesday	Wednesday	Thursday	Friday	Saturday
LIQUIDS							
FOOD							
EXERCISE Type & duration (in mins.)							
PMA 0–10 (positive mental attitude)							
ENERGY 0–10							
Other comments							

ıı 5. Understand How the "Five Ps" Will Teach You a Winning Attitude

The "Five Ps" of Success

The five "Ps" of success are patience, persistence, planning, positive thinking, and perspiration.

Patience is imperative. There are no quick fixes. Contrary to many weight-loss advertisements, the mantras of most of our success stories are more like these: "I'm the tortoise that beats the hare"; "It's a marathon, not a sprint"; "I'm the little engine that could"; and "LSD" (long slow distance). When you stop to think about it, almost anything worthwhile in life—for example, raising a family, reaching educational or professional goals, or establishing a comfortable home—requires patience. In a society that focuses on instant gratification, this can be a difficult concept to master.

Persistence is the essential companion to patience. It is inevitable that in the next 52 weeks of your program, you will have some slumps and unexpected obstacles that may temporarily sidetrack you. Researchers report that the abstinence violation effect (AVE) is one of the leading causes of failure to follow through in weight-management programs. In plain language, this means that when people hit a snag or get off track, they quickly become discouraged and think, "Here I go again, another failure," and tend to quit. On the other hand, we have seen the key to success is not perfection, because we are all human beings dealing with many issues in an imperfect world. The keys are persistence and resilience! So when you experience the inevitable bad day with your program, take a big, slow, deep breath and remind yourself that you are not a computer, a robot, or a saint. Setbacks happen to everyone. The important point is how you react to a setback. Remind yourself that while you are participating in this program you have new tools and resources, and by getting back on track tomorrow you can still succeed and reach your goals. Remind yourself that if you have 25 strong days on your program in the next 30 days, you will have a successful month. In looking at the larger picture, if you have 48 successful weeks out of the next 52 weeks, you will be pleased and excited in regard to your body and health one year from now. If you are persistent, the law of averages will work for you. U.S. president Calvin Coolidge said it well: "Nothing in the world can take the place of persistence. Talent will not; nothing is more common than unsuccessful men with talent. Genius will not; unrewarded genius is almost a proverb. Education will not; the world is full of educated derelicts. Persistence and determination alone are omnipotent. The slogan 'Press On' has solved and always will solve the problems of the human race."

Planning is essential to success. For years when I struggled with my own weight, I can remember saying many times that I would try to be good. Until these good intentions were translated into definite plans, however, I was not able to succeed. With planning, you can implement your program on trips, during the holidays, at work, and so forth. Without planning, you are not likely to succeed. Enjoy the following account by one of our patients as she tells how planning helped her overcome panic concerning an upcoming cruise and how she enjoyed herself without any unwanted weight gain.

Panic over a Cruise
Turns into Smooth Sailing

I've been Dr. Rigden's patient for weight loss for the past six months, and I have already lost around 70 pounds. When my 35th wedding anniversary cruise was approaching, I panicked about keeping my weight stable. I had heard horror stories about gaining weight on cruises. Dr. Rigden assured me, in a calm way, that I simply needed a plan. He said that he had managed to get through a cruise and I could do the same. With constant reminders, pep talks, and strategies from the doctor and his staff with each visit before I left for the Baltics with my husband, I began to feel more confident. I had a plan—and it worked. Over the three-week period that included my 12-day cruise, I lost 6 pounds. Here's how I did it:

- *I read Dr. Walter Willett's book* Eat, Drink and Be Healthy *on Dr. Rigden's recommendation. I even brought it on the cruise as a reference.*
- *I packed my meal replacement shake and a hand mixer, which I used for one or two meals each day (despite the "free" buffets).*
- *I focused on the fun aspects of the cruise, rather than the food,*

and I walked everywhere, including taking the stairs aboard ship instead of the crowded elevators.

- I anticipated the gourmet evening meal each night. The first night at dinner I instructed the waiter that I chose not to have any sauces on my fish or vegetables. The staff was eager to please and always brought me extra steamed veggies with my meals. The food was delicious and I didn't feel "deprived" in any way.
- Yep—I did indulge a few times. When I chose to include dessert after dinner, I ordered one, took the first bite, then passed it to my husband (or around the table).
- At the breakfast and luncheon buffets, I brought my shake (or got a salad) and took extra whole fruits for snacks between meals and when touring off the ship.
- The special late-evening buffets were excellent opportunities to have a cup of decaf cappuccino and fresh fruit. It was a nice treat after dancing.
- Before boarding airplanes I either made a shake or purchased a nice large salad and always had extra fruit.

Dr. Rigden's plan worked! I felt empowered and in control of myself and loved the travel and cruise. Planning ahead paid off (in pounds).

Positive thinking is essential. As you battle over the next 365 days, there will be inevitable challenges that you will need to frame positively. Learn to see the glass of water as half-full instead of half-empty. A typical example occurred yesterday during the appointment of one of our patients. She explained that at work her coworkers were eating cinnamon rolls and she was eating an apple. At first she started to feel sad, but then she began to think positively and framed the experience in a positive format. She reminded herself how excited she was over the benefits of eating differently, including the positive changes to her energy, appearance, and health. She reflected on how poorly she used to feel at work an hour or two after eating foods high in sugar.

In real life, there is no question that sometimes things do not go the way we plan. The following verse, by an unknown author, clearly states the approach we need to use in order to succeed in reinventing ourselves in the face of inevitable adversity.

Don't Quit

When things go wrong, as they sometimes will,
When the road you're trudging seems all uphill,
When the funds are low, and the debts are high,
And you want to smile, but you have to sigh,
When care is pressing you down a bit,
Rest if you must, but don't you quit.

Life is queer with its twists and turns,
As every one of us sometimes learns;
And many a failure comes about,
When you might have won had you stuck it out.
Don't give up though the pace seems slow,
You may succeed with another blow.

Success is failure turned inside out,
The silver tint of the clouds of doubt,
And you never can tell how close you are,
It may be near when it seems so far;
So stick to the fight when you're hardest hit,
It's when things seem worst,
That you must not quit.

— author unknown

Perspiration is an essential element, whether the word is taken literally or metaphorically. We will discuss the role of exercise more fully in another chapter; however, it is essential to your long-term health and well-being whether you have a weight issue or not. Research overwhelmingly conveys that regular, moderate exercise is the leading predictor of successful long-term weight maintenance. Perspiration as a metaphor for the work ethic is also appropriate. Reaching your goal will require hard work and focus, mentally, emotionally, and physically. Interestingly, most of my patients have been very successful in other areas of their lives and have already demonstrated the work ethic, so this is a

The Five "Ps" of Successful Weight Management

1. patience
2. persistence
3. planning
4. positive thinking
5. perspiration

just a reminder. The same philosophy that has helped you to succeed as a teacher, lawyer, home manager, parent, or student applies equally to the area of weight management.

You may be inspired by the following story one patient told about the way she used the five "Ps" to succeed with a difficult weight problem she had endured for 40 years.

Anita's Story:
The Cavewoman Diet Made Me a New Woman

Weight has been my enemy all of my adult life. I was the middle child between two sisters who are both 5 inches taller than I am, and they were overweight as children. My sisters and I always joked about how our parents saw us as one child. We shared one bike, one wagon, one pair of skates, and one radio. Because I was a part of my mother's loving but myopic point of view, I too was convinced that I had a weight problem. According to the weight charts, I was on the high end of normal, but not overweight. We often kidded about our "large bones."

Needless to say, I was shocked when I was measured for bone size and discovered mine were indeed "large." We never lose our childhood impressions. What we were told or believed as children never seems to leave us.

My weight problem began like that of most women, following the birth of my first child, and it got worse with the subsequent births of two more children. In my mid-thirties I decided it was time to face this demon and lose weight. I found a diet on a TV talk show that would let me eat all the protein I wanted. I thought it sounded great— just the stuff I love. Six months later and 60 pounds lighter, I was back to my pre-pregnancy weight.

Of course I could not continue to eat just protein the rest of my life. Through personal stress and the demands of three small children, I let my guard down and the weight came back. All the information about diets foretells that you will eventually gain the weight you lost plus more. Well, I did not want to disappoint the statisticians, and I gained back 70 pounds! I have a wonderful husband who truly loves me, fat or thin. He has been thin his whole life, but he seemed to understand the heartbreak I was experiencing. He gave me the bonus he earned for perfect attendance at work, and I enrolled in a diet clinic. Now, I thought, this was going to be the answer. Everyday one-on-one counseling—who could ask for more? With someone checking on me every day, I lost 72 pounds in six months. I spent all my extra money (there wasn't a lot) on new clothes and makeup. My three kids were grown by now. My daughter (she is 6 inches taller than I am) and I could even share some clothes.

I felt I could do this; I could keep the weight off. However, as soon as I started to increase my calorie intake from the 900 calories I had eaten every day and no longer had my daily pep talks, the old problem came back. I tried all kinds of techniques without success, including cutting back, eating less, buying a smaller plate, and making eating a special occasion. I am no good at counting anything, whether it's calories or stitches on a knitting needle. All I achieved was frustration! During all this weight gain, I suffered arthritis pain in my right hip for eight years. My knees, feet, everything hurt, every day. Not one doctor suggested that I lose weight until six years ago, when a doctor prescribed Phen-Fen. I was lucky. I stayed on that product for only a month. I finally had my hip replaced and my gallbladder removed. Now my genes were rearing their ugly heads. My Mom had had her hip replaced, and my Dad had lost his gallbladder. What next? My Mom had suffered with diabetes since she was just about my age. The test found I was not yet in danger of getting the disease, although my body type (the famous apple shape) and my genes indicated it was highly likely in the near future.

When I began feeling most desperate, a girl at work suggested that I see Dr. Rigden. She brought me his pamphlets. I called and started my visits with the doctor. He ran tests and suggested that I start his Cavewoman Diet for people with Syndrome X (also known as metabolic syndrome, or insulin resistance disorder). I had never had a doctor tell me there was something wrong with me and that weight loss just might be the answer to the problem. At this point in my life, I needed a lifestyle program, not a diet. I needed a way to eat that would fluctuate very little, one that I would be able to stick to for the rest of my life. I am a compulsive eater; make no mistake. I still cook my husband's meals and bake him his favorite coconut custard pie and cornbread. We still buy cookies and the candy he likes. Most of the time I ask him to hide the stuff if I know I will not be able to resist, and there are times when I can't. But I bought two things that I think have helped me more than anything—a mirror (oh, how I used to hate them) and a good scale. (It would take me months to get up the courage to get on my old one.) I placed the mirror right by the bathroom door, so I had to see myself many times during the day. I bought a digital scale (a little pricey, but I don't have to adjust it every time I use it), and I weigh myself every day just before I take a shower. Because of the type of food I was able to eat, Dr. Rigden's food plan is one I can live with the rest of my life. I often joke, "I wish I knew that was my last dish of ice cream. I would have been more selective and enjoyed it more!" I started the food plan "cold turkey" and have had great success. In the past 18 months I have lost 82 pounds and am hoping to lose 20 more. Now my compulsion seems to be buying clothes. It is expensive, but what a great trade-off! I feel younger than I have in years. I walk every day with my husband. And I have more energy than I know what to do with. My test results have been great, and I think that together the doctor and I have saved my life. If you have battled your weight for years, this might just be the place for you. Just ahead is a new life and a wonderful feeling of self-worth.

(I want to thank Anita for her willingness to share this wonderful clinical history with others. Even though she had little or no success battling significant obesity for almost 40 years of her adult life, she has experienced a major breakthrough, employing unbelievable persistence and hard work.)

6. Walk Regularly

Imagine that you are visiting a new doctor for the first time and he is offering you a new medication. Your doctor says this "pill" has incredible benefits that include the following:

- weight loss
- loss of inches of girth
- improved circulation
- stronger heart and lungs
- better blood sugar control
- improved cholesterol, triglycerides, HDL, and LDL
- sharper cognitive function
- reduced stress
- decreased appetite
- increased fat metabolism
- antidepressant effects

Moreover, the doctor informs you this "pill" is *free* and has no side effects. Would you want to take this "pill"? Of course you would!

You have probably guessed that this "pill" and its benefits are all research-proven benefits of regular walking and other moderate, consistent forms of aerobic exercise.

You will be hearing much more about regular, moderate exercise in Chapter 3. Regular exercise is the single most powerful predictor of successful long-term weight maintenance after weight loss. So we might as well get started today!

Jean's story, which follows, illustrates how a previously sedentary, overweight 70-year-old woman can dramatically improve her weight and associated problems by integrating a regular 20-minute daily walk into her lifestyle.

What Is Your Exercise I.Q.?
TRUE/FALSE

1. An example of aerobic exercise is playing softball.
2. Working around the house and in the yard is a good way to burn off calories and fat.
3. A person in good physical condition should exercise to 100 percent maximum heart rate.
4. A moderate, consistent walking program of 30 minutes a day can burn off as much as 16 to 18 pounds of fat in a year.
5. The target heart rate for an overweight patient who has a poor fitness level is 70–85 percent of maximum heart rate.
6. Aerobic exercises, by definition, are continuous for at least 20 minutes and increase the respiratory and heart rates.
7. After 20 minutes of bicycling, if the target heart rate is not reached, it is best to increase speed (intensity of pedaling effort).
8. Exercise can cause physiologic changes in the body that help a person cope with stress and depression.
9. Patients with orthopedic problems in the lower extremities should not exercise.
10. One of the most important strategies to prevent relapse weight gain is to participate in moderate, consistent aerobic exercise.

Answers: 1. false; 2. false; 3. false; 4. true; 5. false; 6. true; 7. false; 8. true; 9. false; 10. true

Jean's Story

Walking Away the Weight

By age 70, Jean had a long-standing history of refractory obesity, hyperlipidemia (elevated cholesterol and triglycerides), and hypertension. She was taking medications for her blood pressure and for elevated cholesterol and triglycerides. However, she had to discontinue her statin drug because of its severe musculoskeletal side effects. Exercise was not a part of her lifestyle.

Jean's Initial Evaluation

Height: 5 feet, 6 inches
Weight: 203 pounds
Waist circumference: 38.5 inches
Blood pressure: 132/66 (nl: 130/80)
Cholesterol: 255 (nl: 180)
HDL: 62
LDL: 147 (elevated, with desirable below 100)
Triglycerides: 232 (nl: 150)
Fasting blood sugar: 105 (nl: 100)

Recommendations

Jean began a 1,400-calorie, low-glycemic-index diet with two scoops of a low-glycemic-index soy-based protein powder each morning, along with daily 20- to 25-minute walks.

4-Week Follow-Up

Jean weighs 193.8 pounds, her blood pressure is 139/85. (Total weight loss: 9.2 pounds)

8-Week Follow-Up

Jean's weight is 189.2 pounds with a blood pressure of 127/61. Her lab work showed a fasting blood sugar of 99, triglycerides of 152, cholesterol 185, HDL 52, and LDL 103. (Total weight loss: 12.8 pounds)

16-Week Follow-Up

Jean feels great and looks forward to her daily walk. Her blood pressure is 135/77 and her weight is 186.4 pounds. Lab work shows a cholesterol of 183, triglycerides of 156, HDL 53, and LDL 99. (Total weight loss: 15.6 pounds)

24-Week Follow-Up

Jean's weight is 182.2 pounds. Her blood pressure is 126/62, and she feels great. (Total weight loss: 19.8 pounds)

36-Week Follow-Up

Jean has a blood pressure of 128/72 and her weight is 179.4 pounds. Her fasting blood sugar is 90, cholesterol 168, triglycerides 109, HDL 56, and LDL 90. She faithfully walks every day! She has lost a total of 22.6 pounds.

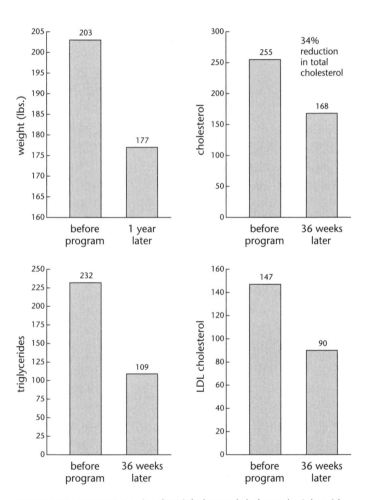

FIGURES 2.1 THROUGH 2.4. Jean's weight loss and cholesterol, triglyceride, and LDL cholesterol reduction

One-Year Follow-Up
Jean's weight is 177.4 pounds.

Summary
Jean has lost 24.6 pounds, lowered her triglycerides 123 points, improved her fasting blood sugar by 16 points, and dropped her LDL 57 points; her total cholesterol has plummeted 87 points.

	INITIAL	FINAL
Weight	203 pounds	177.4 pounds
Fasting blood sugar	106	90
Cholesterol	255	168
Triglycerides	232	109
HDL	62	56
LDL	147	90

7. Don't Forget the Water!

Perhaps the most overlooked part of a weight-management program is optimal water intake. How much water each individual needs can vary. An appropriate water intake depends on where you live, how active you are, and how much you weigh. Overweight people, especially those who are exercising in a warm climate, may require 80 or more ounces a day. Unfortunately, soft drinks, tea, and coffee drinks don't do much to replace the water we lose. Some physiologists estimate that on any given day, half of overweight adults are mildly dehydrated. Whether a person is overweight or not, adequate water consumption is a great idea. It helps the liver metabolize fat, flushes the kidneys and bladder, helps control appetite, and helps maintain muscle tone. It is also essential to help the body eliminate excess sodium and fluids, the retention of which can cause edema and fluid weight gain.

> The most overlooked part of a weight-management program is optimal water intake. Most overweight people need to drink at least 64 ounces of water a day.

Stop Sign Technique

All of us have had a day like the following. You start the morning focused and positive about your program. After a stressful day at work, however, three successive drivers cut you off on the freeway on your commute back home. You make a quick stop at the supermarket. As you wait in the 10-item-only checkout line, someone pushes in front of you with 30 items and numerous redeemable stamps and coupons. Immediately after arriving home, you have to deal with a phone solicitor. All of a sudden you feel yourself hurtling down the slippery slope of inappropriate eating and the old habits start kicking in. What can you do to snap out of it and regain eating "sanity"?

The answer is the Rigden "Stop Sign Technique." First, take out your stop sign and lift your right hand high. Then with vigor slam your hand down on the table and yell loudly "STOP!" Didn't that feel good!? You have just given yourself a conscious shock, a real wake-up call. Second, take three deep slow breaths, exhaling slowly after each one. Third, get very busy with an activity that takes your mind off eating for 20 minutes. During this 20-minute interval, the kitchen or any other food-related areas are off limits.

The Three Steps of the Stop Sign Technique

1. Slam your hand on the table and yell, "STOP!"

2. Take three deep, slow breaths.

3. Get very busy and avoid the kitchen and food-related areas for 20 minutes.

Aldosterone

Aldosterone is a hormone your adrenal glands secrete when you are not drinking enough water. The body has an elaborate negative feedback loop that prevents you from becoming dangerously dehydrated when you are ill, have a fever, or really do not have access to water. When water intake is insufficient, this feedback loop sends signals to the adrenal glands to release aldosterone. This hormone, in turn, causes you to retain fluid and sodium. This is an uncomfortable and frustrating tendency that many overweight patients experience on a daily basis, and they do not understand the root cause. Instead of drinking more water, which turns off the release of aldosterone and allows a vigorous natural diuresis, they instead take diuretics. Unfortunately, these pills just cause further dehydration and perpetuate the body's perceived need to keep releasing aldosterone. The worst-case scenario is combining inadequate water intake with other adverse conditions. Examples include hormonal imbalances during certain times of the menstrual cycle and perimenopause, numerous common medications that cause sodium and fluid retention, and crash diets with too little protein intake. These situations can synergize with aldosterone release to further aggravate chronic edema, a fluid weight gain problem. Assuming normal kidney function and a low sodium intake, the way to have a natural diuresis and remedy this problem is to drink more water!

Since most of our patients come to us when they are only drinking 12 to 16 ounces of water a day, we gradually increase their intake of water to 64 ounces a day.

Carbohydrate Sensitivity

ıl Carbohydrate Sensitivity Screening Questionnaire

Circle the number of any statement that applies to you.

1. I eat out 10 or more times in a week.
2. I consume 14 or more alcoholic drinks in a week.
3. I seldom eat more than two servings (combined) of fruits and vegetables daily.
4. I consume more than 20 ounces of soft drink daily.
5. I seldom exercise 60 minutes or more in a week.
6. I consume refined sugar/carbohydrates at least several times daily.
7. I frequently eat between meals.
8. I consume foods such as hamburgers, hot dogs, pizza, fried chicken, fries, or chips almost every day.
9. I have a problem with stress eating or compulsive eating.

Answer Key: If you have circled four or more statements, your lifestyle and genetics have probably combined to create carbohydrate sensitivity as a major factor in perpetuating your weight problem and keeping you from succeeding in a weight-loss program. It is imperative that as part of your program you carefully evaluate and implement the ideas in this chapter.

ıll Glossary of Medical Terms Used in Chapter 3

aerobic exercise: Aerobic exercise involves the consumption of oxygen. These exercises are continuous and rhythmic, they improve the heart and lungs, and they stimulate fat burn-off. Examples are walking, jogging, biking, and swimming.

carbohydrate sensitivity: A tendency for some people to react to simple carbohydrates such as processed white bread, sugar, white potatoes, or refined grain cereals with an exaggerated release of sugar into the bloodstream after eating; this in turn provokes the body to release extra insulin to help the body to process the blood sugar.

glycemic index: Measures the speed at which you digest food, mainly carbohydrates, and convert it to blood sugar (glucose); the faster the food breaks down, the higher its rating on the index.

isometric exercise: Resistance exercises that increase strength and tone muscles. These exercises include weight-lifting, either with free weights or using weight machines, or exercises that use the weight of the body for resistance.

Mediterranean diet: This is a very healthy diet, much studied by researchers, that is consumed by the inhabitants of southern France, Italy, Greece, and other countries in the Mediterranean region. It is associated with longevity, very little obesity, and far less diabetes and heart disease than we see in the United States. It is characterized by the consumption of relatively large amounts of vegetables and fruit, heart-healthy fats, and low glycemic dietary choices in general.

paleolithic diet: The type of basic, low glycemic diet eaten by our ancestors in the Stone Age (paleolithic period).

SPPMRP: The Soy Protein Powder Meal Replacement Program is an extremely successful program for patients with carbohydrate sensitivity. In essence, it involves two soy protein meal replacements, two to three

low-glycemic snacks, and one low-glycemic meal. The soy protein powder is a very high quality, low-glycemic product that provides excellent
levels of protein, vitamins, and minerals.

systolic and diastolic blood pressure: The top number of the blood pressure 120/80 reading is the systolic blood pressure. It is the pressure in
your arteries when your heart is beating. The bottom number is the diastolic pressure, the pressure in your arteries when your heart is resting
between beats. So, in this example, 120 is the systolic blood pressure and
80 is the diastolic blood pressure.

target heart rate: Maximum heart rate is the number of times per minute your heart pumps when it is working at 100 percent capacity. Never
exercise at your maximum heart rate. Knowing your maximum heart
rate will help you calculate your target heart rate, the number of beats per
minute your heart should pump during aerobic exercise. In general, if
you are relatively fit, your target heart rate should be 70 to 85 percent of
your maximum heart rate. However, if you are in a poor state of fitness
and more than 20 pounds overweight, your initial target heart rate should
be 60 to 70 percent of your maximum heart rate. Reaching your target
heart rate indicates your body is receiving maximum cardiovascular and
fat-burning benefits.

ıl What Is the Significance of Lifestyle?

If you are having difficulty understanding how your lifestyle—in
combination with your unique genetics—could be altered to produce better health and weight results, you don't need to apologize.
Welcome to the club! According to a recent article in the *Journal of
the American Medical Association,* obesity increased in every state of
the country in the 1990s. Physical activity increased in only 11 states
during the same period.[1] One sad fact is that the average American
consumes 35 to 38 percent of his or her total calories as fat, much of
it in the form of harmful trans and saturated fats. High-glycemic-
index foods—that is, foods with high sugar content and minimal nutritional value—make up 20 percent of the average American's diet.
This includes the 40 gallons of soft drinks the average person consumes annually, along with 68 pounds of simple sugars from high-
fructose corn syrup sweeteners. Dr. Walter Willett of the Harvard
School of Medicine, Department of Nutrition, has written, "Genetic

and environmental factors, including diet and lifestyle, both contribute to cardiovascular disease, cancers, and other major causes of mortality, but various lines of evidence indicate that environmental factors are most important."[2] Unfortunately, millions of Americans have not learned what makes up a healthy lifestyle, having been exposed only to a few basic courses in school or to hurriedly given advice from their physicians. In a 2003 study of 6,712 people, published in *The New England Journal of Medicine*, researchers found that only 18 percent of patients received the appropriate counseling and health education that form the cornerstones of effective dietary and lifestyle interventions. This chapter will concentrate on key aspects of your lifestyle that, in combination with your unique genetics, contribute to *carbohydrate sensitivity* and, consequently, switched metabolism.

ıl What Is Carb Sensitivity?

"Carb-sensitive" people, after consuming simple carbohydrates and sugars, experience a rapid spike of blood sugar that triggers, in turn, a spike in insulin and associated metabolic cellular messengers and leads to two negative consequences: the body receives the signal to store, not burn, fat; and the spike in insulin causes a rapid drop in blood sugar; this in turn creates uncomfortable symptoms like fatigue, irritability, headaches, and brain fog. These symptoms stimulate the individual to seek even more carbohydrates and sugars to remedy the uncomfortable feelings associated with the rapid drop in blood sugar.

> When blood sugar drops, a carb-sensitive person can feel an almost desperate need for a pick-me-up and will make statements like, "I crave carbohydrates," "I feel as though I am addicted to sugar," and "I would kill for a quick blast of sugar."

Carb-sensitive overweight people have switched metabolism, a concept we discussed in Chapter 1. After consuming carbohydrate foods with a high-glycemic-index, they have an exaggerated blood sugar and insulin response that causes preferential storage of consumed calories as fat. They do not have metabolic syndrome, hyperinsulinemia, insulin resistance, or diabetes.

There is no consistent test that identifies people with carbohydrate sensitivity, and it is seldom considered or recognized in medical settings. As a result, there are millions of overweight people who are gaining weight rapidly because of this unrecognized metabolic impairment, yet they are nevertheless considered healthy! **It is critical to understand that a person does not go directly from a normal weight-loss metabolism with appropriate blood sugar and insulin physiology to the medical diagnosis of metabolic syndrome** (see Chapter 4). Carbohydrate sensitivity usually develops over a long period of time, as the obese individual slowly transitions from a normal metabolism to insulin resistance. The good news is that carbohydrate sensitivity can be reversed and normal blood sugar and insulin physiology can be restored.

The combination of genetics, lack of exercise, and a diet high in sugar and carbohydrate foods can combine to cause carbohydrate sensitivity.

ıl A New Understanding of Metabolism

In his article "Triglycerides and Toggling the Tummy," C. Kahn explains how medical obesity research has moved beyond calorie counting to the consideration of concepts like carbohydrate sensitivity and switched metabolism: "It was only a few years ago that physiologists and physicians believed that the control of body weight was as simple as 'you are what you eat.' In short, weight gain in the form of increased body fat, leading to obesity, would occur when energy intake exceeded energy expenditure, and weight loss would occur when the converse was true…. Whereas the fundamental principle of energy balance, represented by the first law of thermodynamics, is still true, it has become clear that the mechanisms involved in the control of fat mass are extraordinarily complex."[3]

In his article, "The Functional Medicine Approach to Treating Obesity," Dr. Jeffrey Bland points out that the control of body fat and body composition involves more than the application of calorie counting (the first law of thermodynamics).[4] Have you ever wondered why some people can simply control their calorie intake and easily lose unwanted weight, and why others never seem to have weight problems even when they consume extra calories? Carbohydrate sensitivity can describe the frustrated overweight patient who has tried to limit calories but just seems to keep gaining more weight. Many of these individuals have been accused of "cheating" or "lying" about their diets and have deep emotional scars from these judgments. In fact, carbohydrate sensitivity is frequently the answer, because it causes the calories one consumes to be stored for a rainy day that never comes.

ıl Your Genes Make You Eat Like a Caveman

If you are not interested in biochemistry, perhaps you can best understand switched metabolism associated with carb sensitivity by examining the paleolithic diet research, which seems to indicate we are not what we eat but what our ancestors ate. Research from biochemists, geneticists, nutritionists, and anthropologists on what our ancestors consumed 10,000 years ago has confirmed that our ancestors, at that time, consumed no cultivated grains.[5] In other words, no high-glycemic grains with a rapid blood sugar release entered their systems. Instead, their grain intake was small and often sporadic, and the few grains they ingested were low-glycemic or "slow-release" carbohydrates. These caused only a small release of blood sugar and an associated small insulin response. Now, in direct contrast, it is not uncommon for modern Americans to consume six to ten servings of "fast-release," high-glycemic grains or grain-based simple carbohydrates in a single day. This pattern causes multiple releases of blood sugar peaks that lead to significant insulin responses and associated metabolic messenger molecules that tell the body to store, not burn, fat. Research confirms that genetically, we are no different from our ancestors. It is no wonder, then, that many of us cannot handle this radical change in diet and

> Paleolithic diet research indicates many of us do not have the genes and biochemical machinery to process refined grains and simple carbohydrates, such as white sugar, white flour products, and high-fructose corn syrup. Our ancestors never had to deal with these foods.

thusly suffer carbohydrate sensitivity. That is, many of us simply do not have the genes and effective biochemical machinery to process these types of grains that our ancestors never ate. Celeste's story, which follows, illustrates how carbohydrate sensitivity can affect health and weight. Fortunately, Celeste dedicated herself to a successful program to turn the entire situation around.

Celeste's Story

Stressed Out, Overweight, and Exhausted

Celeste, a 34-year-old, married woman, had been experiencing fatigue for two months when she came to our office. Her migraine headaches had been occurring in clusters every two to three months, as well. At a recent community health screening, she discovered that her cholesterol levels were elevated. She had steadily been gaining weight over the past five years, and her body had not responded well to a number of dieting efforts. She was working full-time and also studying vigorously to earn an advanced degree. She frequently had to eat fast food while on the run, so her diet was high in simple carbohydrates and low in fruits and vegetables. Stress eating and an almost total lack of exercise characterized her lifestyle. Her family history was positive for diabetes mellitus and cardiovascular disease.

Celeste's Initial Evaluation

Height: 4 feet, 8.5 inches
Weight: 140.6 pounds
Blood pressure: 113/74
Waist circumference: 35.5 inches
Cholesterol: 222 (nl: 180)
Triglycerides: 156 (nl: 150)
HDL: 86
LDL: 105 (nl: 100)
Fasting blood sugar: 104 (nl: 100)

Initial Assessment

Our assessment included fatigue, obesity with increased waist circumference (often associated with a tendency to insulin resistance), borderline fasting blood sugar (with a goal of less than 100), elevated total cholesterol (with a goal of less than 180), elevated triglycerides (with a goal of less than 150), and a positive family history of diabetes mellitus and cardiovascular disease.

Recommendations

We recommended that Celeste start a 1,200- to 1,300-calorie, low-glycemic-index food plan with the use of a low-glycemic-index soy protein meal replacement powder as a substitute for breakfast and lunch. In addition, she was urged to exercise aerobically five to seven days a week, with an initial goal of 150 minutes per week. For improved blood sugar and insulin regulation, she started supplements, including chromium 200 mcg twice daily, lipoic acid 200 mg twice daily, and EPA/DHA 1 gram twice daily. Policosanol 10 mg daily was recommended to help her lower her cholesterol. She was advised to drink at least 64 ounces of water daily. She was to see her physician once or twice a month for nutrition education, monitoring, and motivation.

4-Week Follow-Up

Celeste has completely embraced the program. She weighs 127.8 pounds. After starting to exercise for 60 minutes five days per week, she describes having "great energy," with a major reduction in headaches. (Total weight loss: 12.8 pounds)

8-Week Follow-Up

Celeste continues to follow her program with great zeal. Her headaches have resolved and her weight is 118 pounds. (Total weight loss: 22.6 pounds)

12-Week Follow-Up

Celeste weighs 112 pounds, and her lab work shows remarkable improvement. Her fasting blood sugar is 71, cholesterol 155, triglycerides 112, LDL 60, and HDL 74. Her waist circumference has decreased to 27.5 inches. (Total weight loss: 28.6 pounds)

28-Week Follow-Up

Celeste weighs 109.4 pounds and continues to feel great. She is eating a balanced, modified-Mediterranean low-glycemic-index food plan and is totally committed to an active lifestyle. (Total weight loss: 31 pounds)

36-Week Follow-Up

Celeste enjoys her new lifestyle and continues to maintain her weight successfully at 108 pounds. Celeste's appearance has changed so much that her father did not recognize her when he picked her up at the airport. In summary, she has lost almost 31 pounds, dropped 8 inches off her waist circumference, and lowered her fasting blood sugar 33 points. Moreover, she has dropped her cholesterol 67 points, triglycerides 44 points, and LDL 45 points. All without medication!

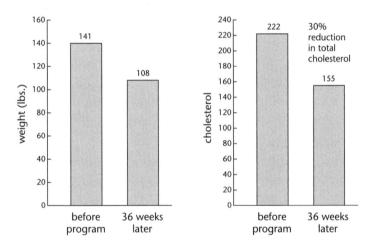

FIGURES 3.1 AND 3.2. Celeste's weight loss and cholesterol reduction

Summary

	INITIAL	FINAL
Weight	140.6 pounds	108 pounds
Waist circumference	35.5 inches	27.5 inches
Cholesterol	222	155
Triglycerides	156	112
HDL	86	74
LDL	105	60

Carole's Story

Carole was an overweight, frustrated 52-year-old woman with a 15-year history of weight yo-yoing when she first came to my office. She had experienced significant weight gain while using antidepressant medication and also attributed some of the weight gain to menopause. In addition to the extra weight, she had low energy and problems with carbohydrate craving. She found that intake of simple carbohydrates (high-glycemic foods) triggered bloating, weight gain, and further craving for these carbohydrates. Just prior to coming to our office, she failed to lose weight after vigorously trying the Atkins Diet.

Carole's Initial Evaluation
Height: 5 feet, 3 inches
Weight: 183.4 pounds
Blood pressure: 128/78
Waist circumference: 39.5 inches
Cholesterol: 246 (optimal below 180)
Triglycerides: 220 (optimal below 150)
HDL: 59
LDL: 164 (optimal below 130)
Fasting blood sugar: 95
Fasting insulin: 15 (optimal below 8)

Initial Assessment
Carole was overweight and was experiencing associated carbohydrate sensitivity, elevated insulin, cholesterol, LDL, and triglycerides. She was undergoing menopause and she experienced low energy and carbohydrate cravings.

Recommendations
We recommended that Carole begin taking the following steps:

1. Start SPPMRP with low-glycemic soy protein powder, two scoops twice daily.
2. Also begin the FMRC Modified Mediterranean diet, 1,400–1,500 calories daily, with five to six small meals.
3. Initiate micronutrient support for blood sugar and insulin regulation with chromium picolinate 200 mcg daily, lipoic acid 200 mg twice daily, and EPA/DHA 1 gram twice daily.

4. Walk at least 30 minutes daily. Keep daily food intake records and drink at least 64 ounces water daily.

Five Months Later

Carole weighs 152.4 pounds. Her other tests and measurements show great improvement, including a waist circumference of 34 inches. Her fasting insulin is 5, triglycerides 69, Cholesterol 198, HDL 31, and LDL 153.

Summary

	INITIAL	FINAL
Weight	183.4 pounds	152.4 pounds
Waist circumference	39.5 inches	34 inches
Cholesterol	246	198
Triglycerides	220	69
HDL	59	31
LDL	164	153

ılı Three Ways to Get Moving

Correcting carbohydrate sensitivity and switched metabolism also requires a commitment to include regular, moderate exercise in your lifestyle.

Physical fitness does not necessarily mean you must participate in 10K races and strenuous aerobics classes. Ideally, we should practice all three of the following types of exercise:

1. **aerobic exercise**—Aerobic exercises increase the body's heart rate, thereby increasing oxygen consumption. These exercises are continuous and rhythmic, improve the heart and lungs, and stimulate fat burn-off. Examples are walking, jogging, biking, and swimming.

2. **stretching**—These activities increase flexibility and keep the body supple. Stretch before and after every walk or workout and when you need to relieve tension in the neck, shoulders, or lower back.

3. **isometrics**—These exercises increase strength and tone muscles and include weight-lifting—either with free weights or using weight machines—or exercises that use the weight of the body for resistance.

Moderate, consistent aerobic exercises are an essential part of any weight-loss or weight-maintenance program. Since most of our adult patients are at least 30 pounds overweight, have not exercised at all for several years, and may have back or lower extremity problems, walking is the most practical exercise choice and is employed by 90 percent of our patients. It is also an excellent choice because it can be continued for a person's entire lifetime and does not require special equipment or clothing. Successful weight management is associated with at least 150 minutes of walking per week, which is about 22 minutes a day or 30 minutes five times weekly. In the weight-loss phase of your program, we recommend at least 75 percent of your exercise be walking or another moderate aerobic activity with isometrics being deferred to maintenance or limited to 25 percent of your efforts. In maintenance, the ratio of aerobic to isometric exercise can be closer to a 50/50 ratio if you wish.

> Successful management of carbohydrate sensitivity and switched metabolism requires at least 150 minutes of walking or other moderate aerobic exercise weekly.

Readers should have a checkup with their physicians before initiating an aerobic exercise program. Any person should avoid aerobic exercise until checking with his or her physician if the following conditions are present:

1. angina (chest pain) at rest or with minimal exertion
2. recent myocardial infarction (heart attack) within three months
3. severe valvular heart disease
4. frequent arrhythmia (irregular beating of the heart)
5. diabetes mellitus that is out of control
6. blood pressure greater than 180/110, even with medication
7. extreme obesity that makes routine walking difficult

8. acute infectious disease

9. resting pulse rate greater than 110

ꟷ Warming Up/Cooling Down

Warming up before aerobic exercise prepares the heart and other muscles for the activity ahead. Warm up for four or five minutes at the beginning of each walk or workout by doing a slower, gentler version of your aerobic activity. Swing your arms and move your body before you start. Cooling down is also important. If you suddenly stop exercising vigorously, your blood pressure can plummet. You could feel weak and dizzy or even pass out. Cool down by performing your aerobic exercise slowly for five to ten minutes, and then by doing some stretches.

ꟷ Don't Overshoot Your Target Heart Range

The resting heart rate is the number of times your heart beats per minute when you are not exerting yourself. In general, the more fit you are, the lower your resting heart rate will be (except for individuals taking beta-blocker drugs, which artificially lower the heart rate). Your maximum heart rate is the number of times per minute your heart pumps when it is working at 100 percent capacity. Never exercise at your maximum heart rate. Knowing your maximum heart rate will help you calculate your target heart rate, the number of beats per minute your heart should pump during aerobic exercise. In general, if you are relatively fit, your target heart rate should be 70 to 85 percent of your maximum heart rate. However, if you are in a poor state of fitness and more than 20 pounds overweight, your initial target heart rate should be 60 to 70 percent of your maximum heart rate. Reaching your target heart rate indicates your body is receiving maximum cardiovascular and fat-burning benefits. Do not be overly concerned if in starting your exercise program you are not able to reach your target heart rate. As you gradually increase the duration and/or intensity of your exercise, you can achieve this heart rate comfortably. Moderate and consistent participation can lead to great things. Do not overdo it, particularly at first.

How to Calculate Your Target Heart Rate

For *moderate-intensity* physical activity, your heart rate should be 50 to 70 percent of your maximum heart rate. For *vigorous-intensity* physical activity, your target heart rate should be 70 to 85 percent of your maximum heart rate.

Your maximum rate is based on your age. To begin your calculation, subtract your age from the number 220. For example, let's say that you are 50 years old:

$$220 - 50 \text{ years} = 170 \text{ beats per minute (bpm)}$$

Your maximum heart rate is 170 beats per minute. According the following formula, moderate-intensity physical activity will require that your heart rate remains between 85 and 119 bpm during physical activity. However, vigorous-intensity physical activity will require that your heart rate remains between 119 and 145 bpm during physical activity.

$$50 \text{ percent level: } 170 \times 0.50 = 85 \text{ bpm}$$
$$70 \text{ percent level: } 170 \times 0.70 = 119 \text{ bpm}$$
$$85 \text{ percent level: } 170 \times 0.85 = 145 \text{ bpm}$$

(Adapted from CDC, "Physical Activity for Everyone" at http://www.cdc.gov/nccdphp/dnpa/physical/measuring/target_heart_rate.htm.)

If your climate precludes comfortable outdoor exercise much of the time, you might want to investigate walking in a mall, purchasing a low-impact exercise video, joining a health club, or buying indoor equipment such as a bicycle or treadmill. In Arizona, where I live, with its very warm and dry weather, walking laps in the shallow end of a swimming pool is popular. Consistent walking is the key, so make it a daily part of life, just like brushing your teeth. Of those who start a walking program, 75 percent of those who exercise in the morning stick with it, 50 percent of those who exercise in the afternoon stick with it, and 25 percent of those who exercise in the evening stick with it.

ıl Get Motivated!

Many of our patients have enjoyed setting up an exercise bank concept. For example, an old shoebox can be labeled "Tom and Sue's Exercise/Vacation Fund." Tom and Sue have pledged to put one dollar in the box every time they walk or work out. Other ideas that link exercise with enjoyable positive outcomes include labeling the box for a birthday, anniversary, or favorite charity. Set up your indoor exercise equipment so you can enjoy a video or television program while exercising. Research has reported that this kind of viewing can create a helpful distraction effect that makes it easier for the exerciser to reach his or her goal. Lively music can certainly be fun and motivating. Look at coordinating your exercise efforts with music that motivates you and gets you moving! Salsa, big band swing, movie themes, Sousa marches, and so on can help keep your energy level high. Listening to an audiobook while exercising can also be an excellent motivational tool. By wearing headphones, a walker can make walking time also "reading time," in a sense, with the option of listening to many different kinds of recorded books. Having an exercise partner can also be a big help, particularly if you are evenly matched in physical capabilities and mutual goals. In fact, many of our patients report walking has improved their relationships because it is an excellent bonding activity.

ıı Pedometers

Many of our patients have embraced wearing a pedometer as a way to monitor their walking progress and provide motivation. A pedometer is inexpensive and gives you immediate feedback. The ultimate goal of wearing a pedometer should be to work up to 10,000 steps daily. This is guaranteed to correlate with good weight-loss results. The following facts explain how pedometers can make a difference:

- The average American logs 5,000 steps, or about two miles, a day.
- When an overweight person logs 10,000 steps per day, it almost guarantees at least a two-pound weight loss in a week.
- One mile is equivalent to 1,000 to 2,500 steps.
- 10,000 steps are roughly equivalent to four to five miles.
- Nine holes of golf without a cart requires 8,000 steps.
- One city block is about 200 steps.
- A 90-minute soccer game requires 8,000 to 10,000 steps.

- The average person walks about 1,200 steps in 10 minutes.
- The average number of steps per day for females, age 30–39, is 5,819.
- The average number of steps per day for males, age 30–39, is 5,162.

ıl Make Daily Activities Part of Your Workout

Increasing physical activity throughout your day should be a daily goal. The ways to accomplish this are limited only by your imagination. A poll taken among our patients yielded the following strategies:

- Take the stairs.
- Stand while on the telephone.
- Put away the remote control.
- Get off the bus one stop early.
- Choose active vacations.
- Avoid using children as "fetch-its."
- Take the long way around.
- Choose outdoor activities.
- Make several trips up the stairs.
- Answer the phone in another room.
- Hand-deliver messages.
- Park farther away from entrances.
- Use a bathroom farther away.
- Go out for entertainment (i.e., museums, fairs).
- Move during commercials.
- Wash the car.
- Set a timer for a short exercise break several times a day.

The following stories show how three overweight patients in different situations were able to succeed in their weight-loss programs by including exercise as an important part of their program. Also, please see endnote #8 on page 225 for comments about case studies typifying our results.

Manny's Story

From Using a Walker to **Being** *a Walker!*

Manny's story illustrates that even a severe physical handicap does
not have to deter an overweight patient from becoming involved
with exercise. At age 62 Manny faced obesity, hypertension, and
severe disability from spinal stenosis and chronic severe degenera-
tive disc disease that required plating and fusion of three discs. He
had borderline blood sugar levels and a fatty liver (steatosis) related
to his obesity. Basic walking and activities of daily living were very
slow, painful, and labored for him. It took great effort for Manny
to walk to the office from his car in the parking lot, often requir-
ing the use of a walker. His family history was positive for diabetes
mellitus.

Manny's Initial Evaluation
Height: 5 feet, 10 inches
Weight: 203.2 pounds
Blood pressure: 128/80
Waist circumference 41 inches
Cholesterol: 226 (nl: 180)
Triglycerides: 128
HDL: 51
LDL: 161 (nl: 130)
Fasting insulin: 19 (optimal below 8)
Fasting blood sugar: 94

Recommendations
In addition to initiating a 1,200- to 1,400-calorie, low-glycemic-
index diet, Manny was advised to take two scoops of a medical food
designed to help correct insulin and blood sugar abnormalities
each morning, along with EPA/DHA 1gram twice daily, chromium
picolinate 200 mcg twice daily, and lipoic acid 200 mg twice daily.

4-Week Follow-Up
Manny weighs 186.6 pounds, his blood pressure is 102/64, and he
feels much better. (Total weight loss: 16.6 pounds)

8-Week Follow-Up
Manny weighs 178.2 pounds with a blood pressure of 102/66.
(Total weight loss: 25 pounds)

12-Week Follow-Up

Even though he has cut his blood pressure medication in half, his blood pressure now is 100/62. He weighs 173.6 pounds and is walking over 2,500 steps some days. (Total weight loss: 29.6 pounds)

24-Week Follow-Up

Manny weighs 170 pounds, and his waist is a 35-inch circumference. His fasting blood sugar is 89, with a fasting insulin of 14. His cholesterol is 190, triglycerides 128, LDL 119, and HDL 50. His blood pressure is 102/60, with further reductions in medication being planned. (Total weight loss: 24 pounds)

32-Week Follow-Up

Manny weighs 171 pounds with a fasting blood sugar of 96, cholesterol 183, triglycerides 88, HDL 61, LDL 107, and fasting insulin of 8.

40-Week Follow-Up

Manny feels great and continues to maintain his weight at 170 pounds.

Regarding exercise, Manny initially was able to walk only 800 to 1,000 steps daily with great difficulty. With resolve and persistence he now is consistently walking 20 to 30 minutes without stopping, with a total of more than 2,000 steps daily in a relatively comfortable manner. His stamina and endurance have greatly improved and enable him to function in a much more independent manner, allowing him to do such things as walk the dog and attend concerts and sports events.

Summary

	INITIAL	FINAL
Weight	203.2 pounds	170 pounds
Waist circumference	41 inches	35 inches
Cholesterol	226	183
Triglycerides	128	88
HDL	51	61
LDL	161	107

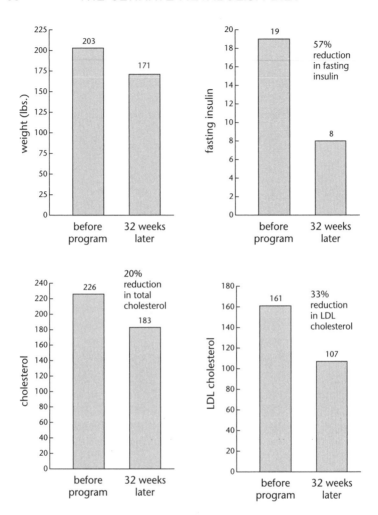

FIGURES 3.3 THROUGH 3.6. Manny's weight loss, insulin reduction, cholesterol reduction, and LDL reduction

Malcolm's Story

Sheds Pounds to Become Award-Winning Rower

Malcolm's story, on the other hand, demonstrates a much more intense involvement with exercise. In his efforts to succeed in managing his weight, Malcolm rediscovered a deep love for athletics that he had experienced in high school and college but had allowed to go dormant. When he came into our office at age 47, he was obese and taking two blood pressure medications as well as two other medications for elevated lipids. He had recently undergone cardiac catheterization to evaluate his chest pains. Due to three leg surgeries, osteoarthritis of the lower extremities, and neck pain due to cervical disc disease, running or jogging was not an option.

Malcolm's Initial Evaluation
Height: 6 feet, 4 inches
Weight: 314.2 pounds
Blood pressure: 142/80 (nl: 130/80)
Waist circumference: 48 inches
Percent body fat: 27.9
Cholesterol: 162
Triglycerides: 193 (nl: 150)
HDL: 35 (nl: 40)
LDL: 95
Fasting blood sugar: 100
Fasting insulin: 45 (nl: 8)

Recommendations
Malcolm began an 1,800-calorie low-glycemic-index diet with the daily usage of a medical food designed to regulate blood sugar and insulin, two scoops each morning, and nutritional supplements including, EPA/DHA 1 gram twice daily, lipoic acid 200 mg twice daily, and chromium 200 mcg twice daily. He chose to try rowing as a new form of regular exercise and completely fell in love with the sport.

4-Week Follow-Up
Malcolm's weight is 308.6 pounds, his blood pressure 128/76, and he is feeling much better. (Total weight loss: 5.6 pounds)

8-Week Follow-Up
At a weight of 299.8 pounds, Malcolm has a blood pressure of 134/76. (Total weight loss: 13.4 pounds)

12-Week Follow-Up
Malcolm's weight is 290.6 pounds, and his blood pressure is 118/76. Previous mild asthmatic symptoms experienced prior to the program have resolved. (Total weight loss: 22.6 pounds)

18-Week Follow-Up

Malcolm has lowered his body fat to 21.7 percent, and he weighs 283.2 pounds. His blood pressure is 118/70. Recent lab tests show cholesterol of 165 and triglycerides 138, HDL 42, LDL 100, and fasting blood sugar 99. (Total weight loss: 30 pounds)

Shortly after starting his program, Malcolm rowed over 200,000 meters between Thanksgiving and Christmas, receiving an award and certificate from a national rowing group. In the next eight weeks, he rowed 540,179 meters, putting him in the top 37 percent of rowers in his age class. Eighteen weeks after starting his program, he was able to row 7,515 meters in 30 minutes, an extraordinary feat!

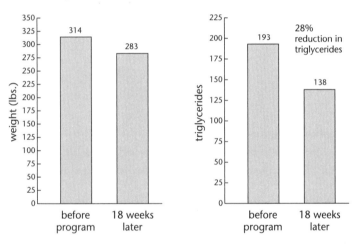

FIGURES 3.7 AND 3.8. Malcolm's weight loss and triglyceride reduction

Summary

	INITIAL	FINAL
Weight	314.2 pounds	283.2 pounds
Waist circumference	48 inches	–
Cholesterol	162	165
Triglycerides	193	138
HDL	35	42
LDL	95	100

ıʅl Treatments for Carbohydrate Sensitivity

The obesity associated with switched metabolism and carbohydrate sensitivity physiologically defends itself and is very difficult to correct. Unfortunately, a traditionally balanced low-calorie, deficit-reduction diet is doomed to fail. We have found that the best results require two dietary interventions. The first is a soy protein powder meal replacement program (SPPMRP), which will break through the sluggish metabolism and provide a much-needed kick-start. Second, a modified Mediterranean diet, also known as the Functional Medicine Research Center (FMRC) low-glycemic-index diet, is introduced for successful long-term maintenance. After I present the SPPMRP, my colleague Barbara Schiltz, RN, MS, CN, will explain the FMRC low-glycemic-index diet. Barb is a codeveloper of these programs. First, however, I would like to explain why I believe these programs work so well.

Two Dietary Interventions for Carb Sensitivity

Phase 1. Soy protein powder meal replacement program (SPPMRP)

Phase 2. FMRC low-glycemic-index diet plan

The SPPMRP features a low-glycemic-index soy-based protein powder that is used to replace breakfast and lunch on a daily basis. (See the Recipes section at the back of the book for more information.) This protein beverage is augmented by two low-glycemic-index snacks and a simple choice of one of four dinner alternatives. This plan has proved invaluable to give the person with carb sensitivity and switched metabolism a simple, streamlined, structured approach that is almost certain to succeed in achieving results right from the start. The food plan is simple, cost-effective, and easy to understand and use. This early success builds confidence and positive momentum and is great for facilitating a transition to a healthier lifestyle and a changed relationship with food. The product our office uses for a low-glycemic soy protein powder is UltraMeal, made by Metagenics Inc. (www.metagenics.com).

While you are losing the first 10 percent of your fat mass on the SPPMRP, this is an ideal time to absorb new nutritional knowledge and an opportunity to integrate new lifestyle habits into your daily routine. The simplicity of the plan is important. My experience has been that at the beginning of a new program, a diversified food plan that offers numerous choices makes success more difficult. It presents the patient with too many opportunities to shoot himself in the foot.

After exhaustive analysis and comparison to many other similar products on the marketplace, I am convinced this meal replacement protein beverage is the best meal replacement protein powder for carb sensitivity–related weight problems. It is composed of the highest-quality soy isoflavone base products on the market. The product has a low-glycemic-index, which improves blood sugar/insulin balance. Its low-fat, soy isoflavone base can help improve cholesterol and provide cardiovascular protection. For example, a meta-analysis of 38 controlled human clinical trials indicates that significant decreases of cholesterol, LDL cholesterol, and triglycerides can be obtained from modest intake of soy protein. The U.S. Food and Drug Administration (FDA) has allowed the following food claim for soy protein: "Diets low in saturated fat and cholesterol that include 25 grams of soy protein a day may decrease the risk of heart disease." The protein beverage we use is unique and superior to other protein powders in that it has been shown by nuclear magnetic resonance studies to cause selective fat loss, not counterfeit muscle weight loss.[6] It also gives the participant a higher probability of success because it provides automatic portion control for two meals a day while the patient is trying to absorb and master complex lifestyle concepts.

ıı Soy Controversy?

Dr. Eleanor Rogan, one of the most highly esteemed researchers in the world on uterine and breast cancers and their relationship to diet, nutrition, and estrogen replacement therapy, presented overwhelming scientific data at the Institute of Functional Medicine meeting in Tampa, Florida, in May 2006. Her twenty-plus years of research indicated that moderate intake of isoflavones from soy was not only safe in terms of breast and uterine cancer, but probably provided some cancer protection. Epidemiological studies clearly show that countries with traditional higher soy intake have relatively low rates of female cancer. There is also much data showing moderate intake of soy may help lessen the effects of PMS and perimenopause. Nevertheless, there have been some speculations in the nutritional field that soy, especially a high intake of isoflavones for many months or years, could potentially cause or provoke breast or uterine cancer. There is absolutely no confirmation of these speculations, which are based on the assumption of very high intake (three or four servings of soy daily) for years. In contrast, our program advocates two servings a day for approximately three months. Nevertheless, if you are still uneasy about using soy in your diet, there are excellent alternative whey-based, low-glycemic protein drinks on the market that are also very effective with this program.

ıı Micronutrients Help Carbohydrate Sensitivity

Although large amounts of data support the concept that micronutrients improve blood sugar and insulin regulation, mainstream medicine by and large refuses to acknowledge these important tools. Micronutrients like chromium, lipoic acid, conjugated linoleic acid (CLA), EPA/DHA, and vanadium are discussed further in Chapter 4.

ıı Phase 1: The Soy Protein Powder Meal Replacement Program (SPPMRP)

Breakfast and Lunch	Mix 2 level scoops of low-glycemic soy protein powder with 8 ounces cold water. Drink this beverage as a meal substitute.
Mid-Morning and Mid-Afternoon Snack	Consume a snack twice daily from the following list: ■ one piece of fruit ■ 12 raw almonds ■ 2 tablespoons of raw seeds ■ 1 piece of whole grain bread ■ 4 ounces low-fat yogurt ■ 1 hard-boiled egg ■ 2 slices of low-fat deli turkey ■ 3 ounces water-packed tuna ■ 1 cup of vegetable, lentil, or legume soup ■ 1 cup fresh tomato-based vegetable juice ■ 1 cup raw vegetables from the low-glycemic vegetable list with ¼ cup salsa

(cont'd.)

Phase 1: The Soy Protein Powder Meal Replacement Program (SPPMRP) (cont'd.)

Evening Meal	One of the following: ■ Large vegetable salad with 4–6 ounces tuna or poultry. You may use 2 tablespoons salad dressing made from equal amounts of canola, sesame, or olive oil with flavored vinegar (i.e., balsamic, raspberry, etc.) ■ Frozen entrée, containing 300 calories and 7 or fewer grams of fat ■ Meatless burrito with one whole-wheat tortilla, ½ cup black beans, ¼ cup brown rice, lettuce, tomato, and ¼ cup salsa ■ 4–6 ounces fish or poultry or 4 ounces lean beef, 2 cups steamed vegetables (nonstarchy, no corn or potatoes), a dinner salad with 2 tablespoons salad dressing made from equal parts of canola, sesame, or olive oil and flavored vinegar (i.e., balsamic, raspberry, etc.)
Supplements	Take a multivitamin daily. If female, take 500 mg calcium citrate daily Avoid the following foods: ■ bread made from refined/low-fiber grains ■ table sugar ■ jam and jelly ■ syrup ■ fruit juices ■ desserts ■ corn (including popcorn) ■ potatoes ■ candy ■ alcohol ■ soft drinks
Drink at least 64 ounces of water daily.	

Vegetables and Fruits on the SPPMRP

Low-Glycemic Vegetables (unlimited servings per day)

■ asparagus	■ artichokes
■ bamboo shoots	■ bean sprouts
■ bell or other peppers	■ broccoli, broccoflower
■ brussels sprouts	■ cauliflower
■ celery	■ chives, onions, leeks, garlic
■ cucumbers/dill pickles	■ cabbage (all types)
■ eggplant	■ green beans

- okra
- snow peas
- sea vegetables (kelp, etc.)
- mushrooms
- radishes
- salsa (sugar-free)
- sprouts
- water chestnuts
- greens: bok choy, escarole, Swiss chard, kale, collard greens, spinach, dandelion, mustard, or beet greens
- lettuce/mixed greens: romaine red and green leaf, endive, spinach, arugula, radicchio, watercress, or chicory
- squash: yellow, summer spaghetti, or zucchini
- tomatoes, tomato-based vegetable juice, tomato juice

Low-Glycemic Fruits (servings limited to two daily)

- apple, 1 medium
- cantaloupe, ½ small
- fresh figs, 2
- grapefruit, 1 whole
- nectarines, 2 small
- peaches, 2 small
- plums, 2 small
- watermelon, 1 slice
- apricot, 3 medium
- cherries, 15 large
- grapes, 15
- honeydew melon, ¼ small
- orange, 1 large
- pear, 1 medium
- tangerines, 2 small
- berries: blackberries or blueberries, 1 cup; raspberries, 1–1¼ cups; strawberries, 1½ cups

ıı Phase 2: The Low-Glycemic-Index Diet (Modified Mediterranean Diet)

In addition to my clinical experience, significant research supports the efficacy of the modified Mediterranean diet, or low-glycemic-index diet plan. Demographic data demonstrate that people in the Mediterranean region are more heart-healthy, live longer, and have far less obesity and diabetes than Americans. The Lyon Heart Study demonstrates that the Mediterranean diet is far more heart-healthy than the American Heart Association diet.[7] In the September 2004 issue of the *Journal of the American Medical Association*, researchers published a study that concluded that "among individuals aged 70 to

90 years, adherence to a Mediterranean diet and healthful lifestyle is associated with a more than 50 percent lower rate of all-causes and cause-specific mortality."[8] It is an interesting diet that our patients have learned to embrace and enjoy.

ıl Introducing Barb Schiltz

Barb Schiltz, RN, MS, CN, has been a valued colleague of mine for the past ten years. She has been a registered nurse for many years and has an undergraduate degree in foods and nutrition and a master's degree in nutrition from Bastyr University. Since 1996 she has worked as a nutrition consultant and research nurse at the Functional Medicine Research Center (FMRC), in Gig Harbor, Washington, monitoring patients undergoing clinical trials for irritable bowel disease, fibromyalgia, diabetes, ADHD, and PMS. Her special interest was expressed in her thesis, "The Unique Role of Carbohydrate Metabolism in Regulation of Glycemic Index." Subsequently, she was instrumental in the development of the low-glycemic-index dietary program for the FMRC. Barb frequently lectures and is a coauthor of articles on topics like managing diabetes and metabolic syndrome with low GI diets, and diagnosing and managing food allergies. She is a gourmet cook who develops healthy recipes and menu ideas. Here Barb shares her expertise on the FMRC low-glycemic-index food plan.

Practical Tips Regarding
the Low-Glycemic-Index (GI) Diet   by Barbara Schiltz

The Functional Medicine Research Center is the research arm of Metagenics Inc. We have been using the low-glycemic-index meal plan for the past eight years with great success. Before we developed this meal plan, I dreaded counseling overweight or obese patients because I became frustrated when most of them gained back their lost weight. Up to this point, my experience proved that almost anyone can lose weight by starving oneself but (in addition to being very unhealthy) it was only a matter of time before a patient would throw in the towel and gain back all the weight that was lost, plus more.

Then came our first clinical trial using this low-glycemic-index meal plan. When the first few patients reported *no hunger* on their follow-up visit one week later, I began to get excited. They explained that they realized they weren't thinking about food constantly. When this experience continued with most of our patients who were following this program, I realized we had struck gold! It was obvious right from the start that the occasional patient who didn't report an absence of hunger or cravings was cheating here and there, often without realizing it (due, for example, to hidden sugars in restaurant sauces or cursory label reading).

Important Guidelines of the FMRC Low-GI Dietary Program

As an overview of this program, the following are the important guidelines to keep in mind:

1. Eat a serving (3 ounces) of fish two to three times a week. If you are a vegetarian, or if circumstances prevent you from eating fish, consume flax oil as a primary fat source. Flax oil is found in the refrigerated section of any health food store. Flax oil and certain types of fish are rich in omega-3 fatty acids, a type of fat that is highly beneficial for helping to restore normal insulin sensitivity.

2. Make sure you consume legumes (beans, peas, lentils) every day. They contain significant amounts of protein and fiber, both of which are important in lowering the blood sugar and insulin response to meals.

3. Eat mixed meals or snacks of protein, carbohydrate, and fat. (Use the sample menus provided in Chapter 4 as a guide.) While carbohydrates eaten alone will often cause an increase in the insulin response, when you eat them as part of a mixed meal, this response is generally lower. The only carbohydrate that may be eaten alone is a piece of whole fresh fruit. The fruits listed in your food plan have been selected because they elicit a low insulin response.

4. Use olive, grapeseed, or canola oil for cooking, and flax oil (with or without olive oil) for homemade salad dressings. These fats favorably impact the ability of your cells to use insulin.

5. Do not consume saturated fat (many cheeses and red meats) or processed foods that include on their labels the words "hydrogenated" or "partially hydrogenated vegetable oils." These fats have a negative effect on the way the body uses insulin.

6. Do not eat starchy vegetables like potatoes and corn (including all types of popcorn), because they cause a rapid increase in blood sugar. (Sweet potatoes and yams are okay.)

7. Do not eat refined carbohydrates/simple sugars (including alcohol, except for small amounts of red wine). Again, these foods cause a rapid rise in insulin.

Table 3.2 lists the basic foods that are emphasized in this program. It is unlikely that these foods will be trigger foods—that is, foods that cause uncontrolled eating or cravings. Eating foods that are low in glycemic index helps to stabilize blood sugar, and thus hunger and cravings should abate.

Table 3.2. Low-Glycemic-Index Food List

Legumes: average serving = ½ cup or as indicated (1 serving = 110 calories)

- yellow and green split peas, or red and green lentils
- beans: garbanzo, pinto, fat-free refried, kidney, black, lima, cannellini, navy, mung
- green soy beans, ⅓ cup
- sweet green peas, ¾ cup
- hummus (¼ cup)
- bean soups, ¾ cup

Nuts and Seeds: serving size as indicated (1 serving = 100 calories)

- almonds or hazelnuts, 10–12 whole nuts
- walnut or pecan halves, 7–8
- cashews, 7–8
- peanuts, 18 nuts or 2 tablespoons
- pistachios, sunflower, pumpkin, or sesame seeds, 2 tablespoons
- nut butter, 1 tablespoon made from nuts listed above

Category 1 Vegetables: (½ cup serving = 10 calories) Servings: Unlimited

- asparagus
- artichokes
- bamboo shoots
- bean sprouts
- bell or other peppers
- broccoli
- brussels sprouts
- cauliflower
- celery
- cucumber
- eggplant
- green beans
- mushrooms
- okra
- radishes
- snow peas
- sprouts
- tomatoes
- water chestnuts, 5 whole
- zucchini, yellow summer, or spaghetti squash

Fruit: (1 serving = 80 calories)

- apple, 1 medium
- apricot, 3 medium
- berries: blackberries or blueberries, 1 cup; raspberries or strawberries, 1½ cups
- cherries, 15
- fresh figs, 2
- grapes, 15
- grapefruit, 1 whole
- kiwi, 2
- mango, ½
- melon: cantaloupe, ½ small, honeydew, ¼ small, 1 slice watermelon
- nectarine, 2 small
- orange, 1 large
- peach, 2 small
- pear, 1 medium
- plum, 3 small
- tangerine, 2 small

(cont'd.)

Table 3.2. Low-Glycemic-Index Food List (cont'd.)

Dairy: average serving size = 6 ounces (1 serving = 80 calories)

- low-fat or fat-free yogurt, plain, 4 ounces (fruit juice sweetened yogurts will also use 1 fruit serving)
- soy milk, low-fat, plain
- milk, nonfat or 1 percent
- buttermilk

Concentrated Protein Sources: (1 serving = 3 ounces at 140–165 calories) Meat, poultry, and fish should be grilled, baked, or roasted (fish can also be poached)

- eggs, 3 egg whites plus 1 whole egg or 2 whole eggs
- egg substitute, ⅔ cup
- fish, including shellfish, 3 ounces fresh, cooked, or ¾ cup canned
- poultry: chicken or cornish hen (breast), turkey, 3 ounces
- leg of lamb, lean cut, 3 ounces
- cottage cheese, low-fat, ¾ cup
- ricotta, part skim or nonfat, ½ cup

- mozzarella, part skim or nonfat, 2 ounces or ½ cup (shredded)
- tofu (fresh), 8 ounces or 1 cup
- baked tofu, 3.5 ounce cube
- tempeh, 3 ounces or ½ cup
- parmesan cheese, 2 tablespoons grated = ⅓ serving
- TVP (soy protein concentrate), ⅓ cup dry = ½ serving

Category 2 Vegetables: (1 serving = 45 calories) Not to be eaten at same meal as whole grains

- carrots, raw, 2 medium or 12 baby, ⅔ cup cooked
- beets, ⅔ cup cooked
- sweet potatoes or yams, ½ small baked

- acorn or butternut squash, ⅓ cup cooked
- rutabaga, parsnips, turnips sparingly

Oils: average serving size = 1 teaspoon or as indicated (1 teaspoon = 40 calories)

- flax seed oil (keep refrigerated)
- expeller pressed olive, canola, grapeseed, sesame oils
- ⅛ avocado

- mayonnaise made with oils listed above
- ripe or green olives, 8–10 medium

Beverages: Servings: Unlimited (0 calories per serving)

Decaffeinated or herbal tea; decaffeinated coffee; water; seltzer, plain or flavored. A modest amount of caffeinated coffee or tea (1–2 cups/day) and wine (1 drink daily) will not disrupt your program. However, for the latter, you should take into account the extra calories consumed.

Condiments: Servings: Unlimited (< 10 calories per serving)

Cinnamon, carob, mustard, horseradish, tamari soy sauce, vinegar, lime, lemon, flavored extracts (e.g., vanilla or almond), herbs/spices

(cont'd.)

Nuts contain "good fats" and are allowed and encouraged, but you should limit yourself to moderate servings of nuts (see chart above) or 1 tablespoon of nut butter each day.

Although legumes contain carbohydrates, they are beneficial carbohydrates that have a low GI and help you feel satisfied after eating them. At least one legume serving a day is important.

Vegetables, of course, contain "good" carbohydrates. It is necessary to eat at least three or four or more daily servings of veggies in category 1 (low GI). You may eat one or two category 2 veggies (medium GI). You must be careful to avoid potatoes and corn, in particular, as they are high GI.

Occasionally we are asked about the higher GI vegetables: rutabaga, parsnips, and turnips. Since these are closer to potato and corn, we suggest you eat only occasional small portions (⅓ cup).

Most fruits contain beneficial carbohydrates, and you may eat them to stave off the hunger and cravings you may have initially. Fruit can help curb sweet cravings. After this period passes, be judicious about fruit. Two to three fruit servings per day are probably best.

Low-fat dairy is consumed as needed. Please adhere to the listed selections. Some lower-fat cheeses are found in the meat category. Although these are certainly dairy products, they contain no carbohydrates, just protein and fat; therefore we consider them concentrated proteins.

Whole grains are a critical food category to control. It may be wise to avoid all grains for the first week or two, if you feel they are trigger foods for you. Some patients feel that being restricted to only one grain is too difficult, and they would rather have none. Others cannot imagine life without grains. Once that period is over, the safest choices are barley, or low carbohydrate tortillas that are available in most grocery stores. They are delicious and usually well tolerated.

Protein is also important to stave off hunger; be sure to eat enough protein foods. Many diet programs have avoided eggs in the past, but they are a healthy and satisfying protein food. Animal proteins that are low in saturated fat are good choices, and so is tofu.

Many people who are struggling with weight issues have traditionally eaten a low-fat diet. However, it is important to have at least four servings of "good fats," (oils, olives, avocado) every day. Salad dressings that contain healthy oils are helpful; however, most prepared dressings also contain high-fructose corn syrup, which must be avoided. A delicious recipe is included in the Recipes section at the back of the book. See Table 3.2 on page 76 for a list of healthy oils.

What foods should you avoid on the low GI diet? Typical high GI foods in the American diet include sugars, artificial sweeteners, white potatoes, corn, beef, pork, and most alcoholic beverages, except for an occasional glass of red wine. Occasional servings of lean cuts of beef and pork may be allowed, but in general beef and pork have a high saturated fat content, which has a negative effect on metabolic syndrome. The refined grains that are not allowed, along with potatoes and corn, all cause a spike in blood sugar and insulin. Table 3.2 also addresses serving sizes. The total number of servings in each food category is determined by the total number of calories you are allowed in your individual program. Also, to help keep your food plan interesting, *please check out my original low-glycemic recipes at the back of the book.*

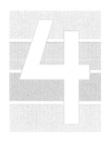

Metabolic Syndrome

ıl Metabolic Syndrome Screening Questionnaire

Circle the number of any statement that applies to you.

1. My family history is positive for diabetes mellitus.
2. My medical history is positive for high triglycerides.
3. My medical history is positive for infertility, unwanted facial hair, or ovarian cysts.
4. I frequently crave sugar and/or carbohydrates.
5. I experience erratic energy and/or mood swings that can be affected by eating.
6. I gain weight in the upper body or have an "apple" body shape.
7. I have experienced gestational diabetes and/or have delivered a baby who weighed more than 9 pounds.
8. My medical history is positive for borderline or confirmed high blood pressure.
9. My medical history is positive for gout and/or elevated uric acid.
10. My medical history is positive for borderline blood sugar readings.

11. My ethnic roots are non-European.

12. I have multiple tiny moles or "skin tags" on my upper body and neck.

Answer Key: If you circled five or more statements, your lifestyle and genomics have probably combined to create metabolic syndrome as a major factor in perpetuating your weight problem and keeping you from success in a weight-loss program. It is imperative that as part of your program you carefully evaluate and implement the ideas presented in this chapter.

ılı Glossary of Medical Terms Used in Chapter 4

acanthosis nigricans: This rash is often associated with metabolic syndrome. It is a dark pigmented rash (usually gray or brown) under the arms or breasts or on the back of the neck.

arcus senilis: This abnormal finding in the eye is often associated with metabolic syndrome. Patients have a white arc or circle around the iris, which ordinarily should only be seen in much older patients.

Caveman/Cavewoman Diet: This diet was developed by Dr. Rigden. It is very effective for breaking insulin resistance and helping patients with metabolic syndrome. It is characterized by large amounts of healthy lean protein, heart-healthy fats, copious nonstarchy vegetables, and low-glycemic fruit.

CRP-hs: C-reactive protein, high sensitivity, is a coronary risk factor that measures the amount of inflammation in the coronary arteries. Inflammation is a problem because it accelerates hardening of the arteries. CRP-hs is often elevated in patients with metabolic syndrome.

glycemic index: Measures the speed at which you digest food, mainly carbohydrates, and convert it to blood sugar (glucose); the faster the food breaks down, the higher its rating on the index.

gout: A painful disorder of the joints, classically involving the foot and especially the large toe. It is very uncomfortable and is caused by elevated levels of uric acid that are deposited in the joints. Uric acid often is elevated in metabolic syndrome.

hirsutism: Unwanted facial hair in females. It is seen in metabolic syndrome and polycystic ovary syndrome (PCOS).

homocysteine: An inherited coronary risk factor in which the patient does not adequately convert the amino acid ornithine to cysteine. The aberrant amino acid produced, homocysteine, can be an abrasive to the inner lining of the arteries, making them more prone to forming plaque. Supplements of B-6, B-12, and folic acid can be helpful in normalizing this situation.

hyperinsulinemia: Refers to having excessive levels of insulin in the bloodstream. Insulin not only regulates blood sugar, it also regulates fat storage. Therefore, hyperinsulinemia tends to promote fat storage and obesity.

insulin resistance: The insulin in the body secreted by the pancreas is not as effective as it should be. Even though the levels of insulin may actually be elevated, people with insulin resistance cannot utilize the insulin. This leads to the pancreas trying to compensate by releasing more and more insulin, which can lead to very negative health consequences like obesity and diabetes.

medical food for insulin management: A nutritional supplement specifically developed to support individuals with insulin resistance and hyperinsulinemia (too much insulin). It is a soy-based protein powder that is low-glycemic and contains high-amylose starch. In contrast to typical starches in the diet, it is slowly broken down and released from the stomach into the bloodstream gradually after ingestion. This leads to a long, slow release of blood sugar, smoothing out the patient's blood sugar and insulin response.

metabolic syndrome: A common cause of obesity in people with the apple-shaped body type; too much insulin in the body, which is not effective because of insulin resistance, characterizes it. These overweight people often have borderline blood sugar, high blood pressure, high triglycerides, and low HDL, and they are generally pre-diabetic.

micronutrients: Nutritional factors in the body like vitamins and minerals that are needed in very small amounts for healthy cellular functioning and metabolism; often they are deficient in patients with metabolic syndrome and these deficiencies are associated with increased metabolic problems. They can be given as supplements and can be an effective part of a program to normalize metabolic syndrome.

polycystic ovary syndrome (PCOS): This condition affects 6 to 10 percent of women of reproductive age. It is the most common cause of anovulatory infertility, in which females have menstrual cycles without ovulation. Seventy percent of PCOS women are obese. Elevated levels of androgen, ovulation problems, and ovarian cysts define it.

skin tags: Small growths located around the neck and upper body that are often associated with metabolic syndrome.

sleep apnea: A sleep disorder, often associated with metabolic syndrome; it is characterized by erratic breathing, often associated with snoring, that compromises oxygenation of the brain during the night. The following day often is characterized by fatigue and sleepiness.

Ivan's Story

Creating a Better Future on the Caveman Diet

By age 46, Ivan was dealing with numerous medical conditions in addition to morbid obesity that had resisted numerous dietary reduction efforts. He was also taking a number of powerful medications for these conditions. His physical examination showed skin tags around his upper body and neck and a dark pigmented rash called acanthosis nigricans under his arms and torso.

Ivan's Initial Evaluation

Height: 6 feet, 1 inch
Weight: 390.3 pounds
Blood pressure: 169/98 (nl: 130/80)
Fasting insulin: 113 (nl: 8)
Two-hour postprandial (after eating) insulin: 121 (nl: 25)

Recommendations

We recommended that Ivan begin taking the following steps:

1. Start a 1,200- to 1,400-calorie Caveman Diet, along with two scoops of a medical food designed to manage metabolic syndrome. After losing 10 percent of his initial weight, Ivan continued with a 1,200- to 1,400-calorie low-glycemic-index diet, with two scoops each morning of the same medical food.
2. Start taking chromium 200 mcg daily, vanadyl sulfate 20 mg daily, conjugated linoleic acid 1 gram twice daily.
3. Initiate a daily 20-minute walk.
4. Keep careful daily records of food and water intake and exercise.
5. Commit to regular visits with his physician for monitoring, patient education, and motivation.

10-Week Follow-Up
Ivan's weight is 362.6 pounds, and his blood pressure is 142/84. (Total weight loss: 28.7 pounds)

20-Week Follow-Up
Ivan's weight is 332.8 pounds, and his blood pressure is 140/76. (Total weight loss: 58.5 pounds)

24-Week Follow-Up
Ivan's weight is 312.4 pounds, and his blood pressure is 143/93, and fasting insulin 20. (Total weight loss: 78.9 pounds)

36-Week Follow-Up
Ivan's weight is 295 pounds, and his blood pressure is 141/87. (Total weight loss: 96.3 pounds)

18-Month Follow-Up
Ivan's weight is 282 pounds, and his blood pressure is 130/94. (Total weight loss: 109.3 pounds)

2-Year Follow-Up
Ivan's weight is 270 pounds, with a fasting insulin of 12.3.

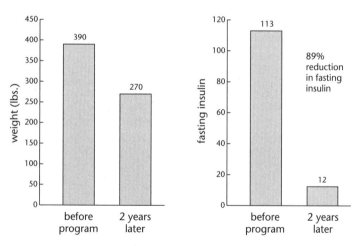

FIGURES 4.1 AND 4.2. Ivan's weight loss and fasting insulin results

Summary
Ivan has just repeated his sleep study. He no longer needs CPAP (a breathing machine used for obstructive sleep apnea) and now has a normal sleep pattern. Furthermore, his skin tags and acanthosis

nigricans are spontaneously clearing. He is walking 3 to 5 miles daily or biking 10 to 12 miles per day. He has cut his medications by more than half. He has lost a total of 121.4 pounds, lowered his systolic blood pressure 39 points, and reduced his insulin by an amazing 101 units. He experienced at least a 50 percent improvement in all of the various symptoms related to his multiple chronic illnesses.

	INITIAL	FINAL
Weight	390.3 pounds	270 pounds
Blood pressure	169/98	130/94
Insulin	113	12.3

ıl What Is Metabolic Syndrome?

In spite of a 20-year emphasis in our society on low-fat and nonfat foods and an overall decrease in fat-calorie consumption, we are in the midst of an epidemic of obesity related to metabolic syndrome (a.k.a., syndrome X, or insulin resistance syndrome). Recent research reports that metabolic syndrome is highly prevalent, expressing in 24 percent of adults, or approximately 60 to 75 million Americans. Moreover, the vast majorities of these adults have associated obesity and remain undiagnosed![1]

Metabolic syndrome is a condition that features the combination of insulin resistance and hyperinsulinemia (too much insulin), which has profound health implications. Presently, the criteria published by the National Cholesterol Education Program Adult Treatment Panel III include five features of metabolic syndrome, three of which must be present to define the syndrome. These criteria are:

1. elevated waist circumference (greater than 40 inches in males and 35 inches in females)

2. triglyceride levels above 150 mg/dl

3. decreased HDL (less than 40 mg/dl for men and below 50 mg/dl for females)

4. blood pressure above 130/85

5. fasting blood sugar above 100 mg/dl

Individuals who suffer from metabolic syndrome have enough insulin to process blood sugar (glucose) well enough to avoid diabetes. Instead, their excessive insulin levels compensate for insulin resistance; insulin resistance is impairment at the molecular level that interferes with the normal ability of the body to transport blood sugar from the bloodstream into cells.

Hyperinsulinemia (excessive insulin) is highly correlated with the increasingly common conditions of obesity, coronary heart disease, hypertension, and diabetes mellitus type 2. There are numerous clinical conditions associated with metabolic syndrome such as breast cancer, gout, and hypertension. Nevertheless, it has been my clinical experience that very few patients I see for the first time have ever undergone an evaluation of their insulin level. These patients are totally unaware of the existence of metabolic syndrome. These circumstances are remarkable when one considers that an insulin blood test is readily available and is covered by insurance. Moreover, most of these patients have had lipid profiles showing elevated triglycerides with low HDL levels. (Their triglyceride/HDL ratios are usually over 4.) This elevated ratio correlates positively with insulin resistance.

Clinical Conditions Associated with Metabolic Syndrome
- obesity
- breast cancer
- hyperinsulinemia
- stroke
- adult-onset diabetes mellitus
- sleep apnea
- polycystic ovary syndrome
- gout
- hypertension
- cardiovascular disease
- hyperlipidemia

As I pointed out earlier, obesity is the leading preventable cause of death in the United States, and the American public is spending more than $100 billion each year on obesity-related health-care costs. Coronary heart disease is the leading cause of mortality and disability in the United States. Hypertension has been estimated to affect more than 50 million people in this country. The American Diabetes Association states that diabetes alone accounts for 178,000 deaths, 54,000 amputations, and up to 24,000 cases of blindness annually. It is estimated that diabetes and its complications account for

$45 billion a year in medical care costs. Since metabolic syndrome is a major precursor to these conditions, the potential health-care cost of metabolic syndrome is enormous.

Metabolic syndrome is caused by the interaction of genetic susceptibility to developing excessive levels of insulin and subsequent insulin resistance combined with placing these genes in nutritional environments and lifestyles that lead to the expression of this syndrome. In an article in the *American Journal of Physiology*, researchers stated that half of the variability of insulin action was due to lifestyle, the other half to the genes. Of the 50 percent attributed to lifestyle, half was due to lack of fitness, half to obesity.[2]

I try to explain this complex interaction to my patients in the following way. The first physiologic change detected in metabolic syndrome is an increase in insulin levels. Besides regulating blood sugar, insulin stimulates messenger molecules and enzymes to regulate fat metabolism. Specifically, high levels of insulin direct the fat cells to hold onto fat and store it, not burn it for energy. This increase of fat deposits and fat storage occurs particularly in the abdominal area. After a critical fat mass is reached, the increased level of stored fat cells creates another problem for the body. The increased fat around body cells produces a kind of insulin resistance, decreasing the ability of the insulin to regulate blood sugar successfully. The pancreas then compensates by releasing more and more insulin until the blood sugar is successfully regulated. Thus, a vicious cycle is created for the person who develops upper body or abdominal "apple" obesity. Excessive insulin secretion, fat storage at the expense of fat burning, the development of insulin resistance related to poor blood sugar regulation, and compensatory pancreatic overproduction of insulin all contribute to this vicious cycle (see Figure 4.3 on the next page).

There are two important consequences of this vicious cycle:

1. The pancreas cannot indefinitely produce two or three times the normal amounts of insulin, so it burns out and diabetes eventually develops.
2. As a consequence of their genetics, metabolic syndrome individuals release large spikes of insulin in response to high-glycemic foods that rapidly release blood sugar into the

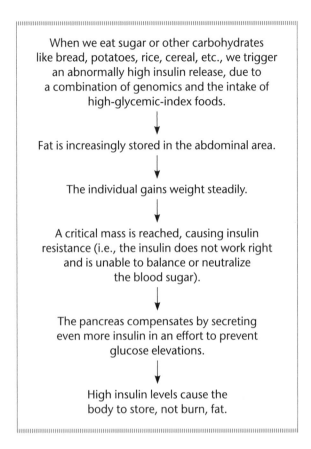

FIGURE 4.3. The vicious cycle of increased insulin secretion, insulin resistance, and obesity

bloodstream. These spikes of insulin can cause rapid drops in blood sugar. As a result, blood sugar levels in these individuals do not decrease smoothly over the next three to five hours as they should. Instead, they tend to plummet downward abruptly, causing symptoms of fatigue, brain fog, irritability, headaches, anxiety, and hunger. Experiencing these symptoms is very uncomfortable to the brain and central nervous system. An emergency signal is released into the body that is interpreted as an immediate need for a pick-me-up snack.

Hazel's Story

Taming Metabolic Syndrome

By age 62, Hazel had been battling obesity for most of her life. During the previous 20 years, she had lost a significant amount of weight in two separate attempts, but had subsequently regained it. She craved sweets and had problems with compulsive eating. She suffered from knee pain, sciatica, and fatigue. Her medical history included a hip replacement and gall bladder surgery. Her physical examination was within normal limits except for a decreased range of motion in her spine and knees, which had hypertrophied.

Hazel's Initial Evaluation

Height: 5 feet, 3.75 inches
Weight: 243.6 pounds
Blood pressure: 138/98 (nl: 130/80)
Waist circumference: 47 inches
Hip circumference: 57 inches
Body fat: 39.7 percent
Cholesterol: 209 (nl: 180)
LDL: 131 (nl: 100)
Fasting insulin: 105 (nl: 8)

Recommendations

We recommended that Hazel begin taking the following steps:

1. Start a 1,200- to 1,400- calorie Cavewoman Diet. After losing 10 percent of initial weight, continue with a 1,200- to 1,400-calorie, low-glycemic-index diet. With both food plans, Hazel was advised to take two scoops of a medical food daily that was designed for the regulation of metabolic syndrome.
2. Take supplements: chromium 200 mcg daily, vanadyl sulfate 7.5 mg daily, conjugated linoleic acid 1 gram twice daily.
3. Walk 150 minutes or more per week.
4. Drink 64 to 100 ounces of water daily.
5. Keep meticulous daily dietary records.
6. Commit to regular physician visits for regular monitoring, education, and motivation.

1-Month Follow-Up

Hazel weighs 233.8 pounds; her blood pressure is 137/93. (Total weight loss: 9.8 pounds)

4-Month Follow-Up

Hazel's weight is 213.2 pounds, her blood pressure is 125/91, and she has a fasting insulin of 9. (Total weight loss: 30.4 pounds)

9-Month Follow-Up

Hazel's weight is 178.2 pounds, her blood pressure is 131/79, and her cholesterol is 196, LDL 112. (Total weight loss: 65.4 pounds)

18-Month Follow-Up

Hazel's weight is 166.2 pounds, her blood pressure is 120/80, her percent body fat is 30.1, and she has a waist circumference of 33.5 inches and a hip circumference of 45.5 inches. (Total weight loss: 77.4 pounds)

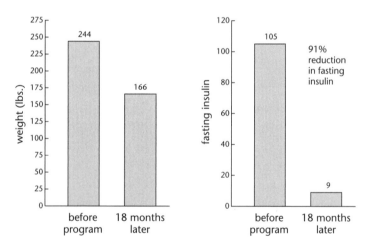

FIGURES 4.4 AND 4.5. Hazel's weight and fasting insulin improvement

Summary

Hazel has lost 77.4 pounds and reduced both her systolic and diastolic blood pressure 18 points each. She has lost nearly 14 inches from her waist, lowered her cholesterol 13 points and her LDL cholesterol 19 points; her insulin has improved by an amazing 96 units.

	INITIAL	FINAL
Weight	243.6 pounds	166.2 pounds
Waist circumference	47 inches	33.5 inches
Cholesterol	209	196
LDL	131	112
Blood pressure	138/98	120/80
Insulin	105	9

ıl Ethnicity and Metabolic Syndrome

There is much evidence that ethnicity plays a role in developing metabolic syndrome. People of non-European origin are at a much greater risk. Classic examples are the Pima Indians, described in Chapter 1, South Asian Indians, Japanese Americans, African Americans, Australian Aborigines, Mexican Americans, and various Pacific Island populations. A number of researchers have published data comparing the Pima Indians in the United States to those in Northern Mexico, who are closely related genetically.[3] Today, nearly 60 percent of the U.S. adult Pima population have type 2 diabetes, and that population has the highest percentage of obese individuals in the world. In sharp contrast, closely related Pima natives in Northern Mexico have not adopted a modern diet, which is high in sugar, salt, fat, and alcohol, nor have they assumed a sedentary lifestyle. The Mexican Pima population has a very low incidence of type 2 diabetes and obesity.

> People of non-European origin are at a much greater risk for developing metabolic syndrome. Examples are the Pima Indians, Japanese Americans, African Americans, Mexican Americans, and various Pacific Island populations.

Type 2 diabetes increases a person's tendency toward obesity. It appears to be a two-way street. Not only does obesity make one susceptible to diabetes, but type 2 diabetes is also associated with the visceral (also called abdominal or "apple") fat distribution pattern. One researcher used the term "thrifty genotype" to explain this tendency in metabolic syndrome, type 2 diabetes, and obesity.[4] In the course of human evolution, according to this theory, those individuals who tended to store fat at an accelerated rate during periods of food abundance would be at an evolutionary advantage and able to survive famine long enough to pass on those thrifty genes to their offspring. Now, in times of abundant food and relatively continuous "feast," individuals with this genetic attribute are much more susceptible to weight gain.

ıl The Relationship of Metabolic Syndrome to Other Conditions

Metabolic syndrome needs to be recognized and treated, not only for its role in obesity, but also as a key causative factor in coronary heart disease, diabetes, and hypertension.

ıl Coronary Heart Disease (CHD)

Hyperinsulinemia has been associated with increased risk for coronary heart disease (CHD). A high insulin level, particularly when fasting, is an independent risk factor for CHD. Insulin stimulates lipogenesis (the manufacture of fatty deposits) in arterial tissue and enhances the growth and proliferation of arterial smooth-muscle cells, leading to the deposit of dangerous plaque. High insulin levels further lead to high triglycerides and depressed high-density lipoproteins (HDL). This combination of high triglycerides and low HDL is another risk factor for CHD. Insulin resistance and associated high insulin levels may also be related to CHD through a condition that causes blood platelets to clump and form clots.

Researchers have recently found that insulin resistance increases the number of cellular adhesion molecules, a condition that makes the endothelium (inner arterial lining) stickier. Insulin resistance also leads to decreased production of nitric oxide, which causes the arteries to constrict and harden. All of these changes promote arterial blockage and inflammation. The linkage between metabolic syndrome and CRP-hs, a marker for coronary artery inflammation, has been clearly established. There also appears to be an association between the cardiovascular risk factor homocysteine and insulin resistance. Clearly, metabolic syndrome is a dangerous condition in terms of cardiovascular risk.

> Elevated insulin levels and insulin resistance are present in metabolic syndrome. These factors increase the onset and development of coronary heart disease by promoting fatty deposits in the coronary arteries, increasing triglycerides, and lowering good cholesterol. They also make the blood thicker and the artery walls more sticky, constricted, and hard. These changes all promote arterial blockage and inflammation.

ıı Type 2 Diabetes Mellitus

Basically, one of two things can happen when the body's insulin system breaks down: The body produces little or no insulin and type 1 diabetes develops, or the pancreas produces an abundance of insulin that the body does not respond to normally, creating risk for either type 2 diabetes or metabolic syndrome. Insulin action varies enormously in normal people. Insulin action may be ten times more efficient in normal people than in the insulin-resistant patient. About 25 percent of the nondiabetic population are just as insulin-resistant as those with type 2 diabetes, and they are at risk of developing metabolic syndrome. The difference between type 2 diabetes and metabolic syndrome can therefore be summed up simply. The key problem leading to type 2 diabetes is insulin resistance coupled with the inability to secrete enough insulin to overcome that resistance. The root of metabolic syndrome, however, is the combination of insulin resistance plus too much insulin, which is released excessively by the pancreas to try to overcome insulin resistance at the cellular level.

> Type 2 diabetes mellitus patients have insulin resistance but not enough insulin to overcome that resistance. In contrast, patients with metabolic syndrome have insulin resistance plus compensatory increased levels of insulin.

In the basic biochemistry of cellular blood sugar/insulin interactions, several nutritional factors have key roles in combating insulin resistance and establishing normal blood sugar metabolism at the cellular level. These factors include EPA/DHA, vanadium, chromium, concentrated linoleic acid, lipoic acid, inositol, magnesium, and vitamin E.

ιι What Happens When Metabolic Syndrome Becomes Diabetes?

Unfortunately, metabolic syndrome not only causes switched metabolism, it is also a prediabetic condition. The following stories of Joe and Hans show how powerful the corrective programs presented in this book can be within a relatively short period of time. By creating a healthier food and lifestyle environment for one's genes with an appropriate low-glycemic food plan, moderate exercise, and medical foods designed to regulate blood sugar and insulin metabolism, one can rapidly reverse and even correct potentially serious medical consequences as well as facilitate weight loss.

(Joe's Story)

Metabolic Syndrome Led to Diabetes Mellitus
Joe came to us because he had been feeling poorly for one to two months, suffering lethargy, urinary frequency, and decreased visual acuity. At age 62, he had not received any medical care for several years. He was not taking any medications, and there was no contributing family history to explain his symptoms.

Joe's Initial Evaluation
Height: 5 feet, 9 inches
Weight: 223 pounds
Blood pressure: 142/86 (nl: 130/80)
Cholesterol: 224 (nl: 180)
Triglycerides: 253 (nl: 150)
HDL: 54
LDL: 178 (nl: 130)
Cholesterol/HDL ratio: 4.1 (nl: 3.5)
Triglyceride/HDL ratio: 4.9 (nl: 4.0)

Fasting blood sugar: 183 (nl: 100)

Fasting blood sugar repeated in 24 hours: 197 (nl: 100)

Joe's blood pressure, cholesterol, triglycerides, LDL, triglyceride/-HDL ratio (which correlates with insulin resistance), and blood sugar levels were all abnormally elevated. The blood sugar values were definitely in the diabetic range.

Initial Assessment

Joe was deemed to be suffering from the following conditions:

1. diabetes mellitus with insulin resistance
2. obesity
3. hypertension
4. elevated cholesterol, LDL, and triglycerides
5. a very high cardiovascular risk and the need for aggressive medical intervention

Recommendations

The patient was given two choices of care: (1) aggressive functional medicine/nutritional-lifestyle intervention; or (2) the initiation of several prescriptions along the traditional medical-care model. The latter would include one or two diabetic medications, medications for cholesterol and triglycerides, and an antihypertensive. If he wanted to choose the functional medicine model, he was informed that he would need to show impressive improvement in six weeks in order to avoid multiple medications and implementation of the traditional medical model. The patient chose the first option.

We then recommended that Joe begin taking the following steps:

1. Initiate the FMRC low-glycemic-index diet of 1,400 to 1,500 calories, involving five to six small meals daily. In addition, start using a medical food designed to regulate blood sugar/insulin abnormalities, two scoops twice daily.
2. Walk 30 minutes daily.
3. Start EPA/DHA 1 gram twice daily, and supplement containing micronutrient support for blood sugar/insulin regulation, one tablet twice daily.

Two Week Follow-Up

Joe's weight is 219.2 pounds; his fasting blood sugar is 126.

Six-Week Follow-Up

Joe's weight is 213.2 pounds, his blood pressure is 138/70, fasting blood sugar 119, cholesterol 150, triglycerides 65, HDL 45, LDL 94, cholesterol/HDL ratio 3.3, and triglycerides/HDL ratio 1.3. The patient feels great.

Seven-Week Follow-Up

Fasting blood sugar is 94.

Joe agrees to long-term follow-up and a commitment to reduce to a weight of 190 pounds or less.

Summary

	INITIAL	FINAL (7 WEEKS LATER)
Weight	224 pounds	213.2 pounds
Blood pressure	142/86	138/70
Cholesterol	224	150
Triglycerides	253	65
HDL	54	45
LDL	178	94
Fasting blood sugar	183, 197	119, 94
Cholesterol/HDL	4.1	3.3
Triglycerides/HDL	4.9	1.3

In just seven weeks, with a weight loss of 11 pounds, Joe was able to normalize a potentially dangerous medical situation and avoid multiple pharmaceuticals. His blood pressure, cholesterol, triglycerides, LDL, fasting blood sugar, and cholesterol/HDL and triglyceride/HDL ratios were all amazingly improved. This shows that he was able to "reinvent" himself metabolically with the help of his specially designed medical food, low-glycemic-index diet, and lifestyle changes.

Hans's Story

Lifestyle Changes Ward Off Diabetes Mellitus

At age 53, Hans came to our office complaining of headaches, dizziness, and high blood pressure. He had mild hypertension that was being controlled with Lisinopril. He also had a history of border-line blood sugar and triglyceride levels. His family history was positive for diabetes mellitus and heart disease. Recently, he had been experiencing high levels of stress and had been consuming excessive carbohydrates and alcohol. His blood pressure at work had been recorded in the 160–170 systolic range on three occasions.

Hans's Initial Evaluation

Height: 5 feet, 11 inches
Weight: 211.6 pounds
Blood pressure: 122/70
Cholesterol: 201 (nl: 180)
Triglycerides: 732 (nl: 150)
HDL: 29 (nl: 40)
Fasting blood sugar: 173 (nl: 100)
Cholesterol/HDL ratio: 6.7 (nl: 3.5)
Triglycride/HDL ratio: 24.4 (over 4 confirms insulin resistance)

Initial Assessment

Hans was deemed to be suffering from the following conditions:

1. diabetes mellitus with insulin resistance
2. overweight
3. markedly elevated triglycerides, decreased HDL
4. hypertension, recent exacerbation, previously well controlled on Lisinopril
5. elevated life stress impacting diet and alcohol consumption

Recommendations

The patient was given two choices of care: (1) aggressive functional medicine/nutritional-lifestyle intervention; or (2) the initiation of several prescriptions along the traditional medical-care mode. The latter would include one or two diabetic meds, a med for triglycerides, and possibly additional hypertension medication. If he wanted to choose the functional medicine model, he was informed that he would need to show impressive improvement in six weeks in order to avoid multiple medications and implementation of the traditional medical model. The patient chose the first option.

We then recommended that Hans begin taking the following steps:

1. Initiate the FMRC low-glycemic-index diet of 1,400 to 1,500 calories, consumed in five to six small meals daily. In addition,

start using a medical food designed to regulate blood sugar/-insulin abnormalities, two scoops twice daily.
2. Walk 30 minutes daily.
3. Start EPA/DHA 1 gram twice a day, and supplement containing micronutrient support for blood sugar/insulin regulation, one tablet twice a day.
4. Stop alcohol consumption, in conjunction with stress-management counseling.

Two-Week Follow-Up
Hans's weight is 204.7 pounds, his blood pressure is 112/72.

Six-Week Follow-Up
Hans's weight is 193.8 pounds, his blood pressure is 118/68, fasting blood sugar 102, cholesterol 154, HDL 22, triglycerides 110, LDL 110, cholesterol/HDL 7.0, and triglycerides/HDL 5.0.

Hans feels much better and agrees to long-term follow-up, committing to achieving a weight of 180 pounds or less, with a normal fasting blood sugar and Hgb A1C levels.

Summary

	INITIAL	FINAL (6 WEEKS LATER)
Weight	211.6 pounds	193.8 pounds
Blood pressure	122/70	118/68
Fasting blood sugar	173	102
Cholesterol	201	154
Triglycerides	732	110
HDL	29	22
LDL	invalid	110
Cholesterol/HDL ratio	6.7	7.0
Triglyceride/HDL ratio	24.4	5.0

Comments
In just six weeks, with a weight loss of 18 pounds, Hans was able to correct a diabetic challenge and show a remarkable drop in his triglycerides. His blood pressure, LDL, and triglyceride/HDL ratio also showed significant positive change. This story illustrates that

the proper lifestyle, diet, and natural supplements tailored to an individual's metabolic needs can have startling results and, in a sense, reinvent one's metabolism.

ıı Hypertension

Doctors have known for many years that patients with hypertension are at a greatly increased risk for heart attack, stroke, or both, whether or not they have metabolic syndrome. Not surprisingly, several large-scale clinical trials have shown that lowering blood pressure will significantly decrease the risk of stroke and fatal heart attack.

Fifty percent of patients with high blood pressure are also insulin-resistant, with increased insulin levels and other manifestations of metabolic syndrome. Research confirms that these patients are at great risk of having a heart attack.

For years, experts have hypothesized that excessive sodium is a major cause of hypertension. It appears that insulin can also influence this tendency. Although insulin does not damage the kidneys, it influences them to retain sodium and fluid. This relationship between insulin and blood pressure is supported by the repeated observation, in our medical practice, that weight loss and lowered insulin levels often normalize blood pressure. In addition, bothersome fluid retention and edema are often corrected. This change frequently occurs with a 10 percent loss of initial mass, and may be seen with just a 5 percent loss. It is a joy to see patients who are able to stop their blood pressure medications safely.

> Fifty percent of patients with high blood pressure are also insulin-resistant, with metabolic syndrome. Weight loss and lowering insulin levels can lead to improved and sometimes normal blood pressure.

ıı Obesity

Lipoprotein lipase is an enzyme that promotes fat storage. Therefore, insulin promotes fat accumulation by activating lipoprotein lipase, which initiates the removal and uptake of triglycerides from blood into fat cells. It also inhibits fat burning by inhibiting hormone-sensitive lipase, an

> Insulin promotes fat storage by activating an enzyme called lipoprotein lipase. It particularly does this in the upper abdominal area.

enzyme that breaks down stored triglycerides into free fatty acids. In other words, high levels of insulin promote the storage of abdominal fat, whereas decreasing levels of insulin helps to promote fat loss. It is important to point out that obesity by itself does not cause insulin resistance. Not all obese people are insulin-resistant and not everyone with metabolic syndrome is obese. The key is the genetics of each individual.[5]

Figure 4.6 (below) summarizes the potentially dangerous relationships of metabolic syndrome to other medical problems.

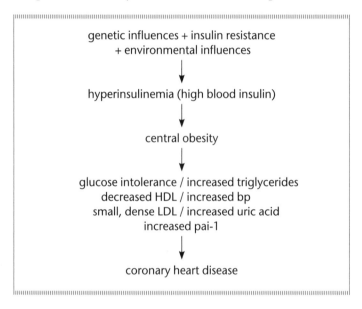

genetic influences + insulin resistance
+ environmental influences

↓

hyperinsulinemia (high blood insulin)

↓

central obesity

↓

glucose intolerance / increased triglycerides
decreased HDL / increased bp
small, dense LDL / increased uric acid
increased pai-1

↓

coronary heart disease

FIGURE 4.6. Physiological relationships of metabolic syndrome

ıll Check the Family Tree for Metabolic Syndrome

Frequently, the metabolic syndrome patient has a family history that is positive for diabetes, obesity, hypertension, and heart disease. Personal medical history may include large babies, gestational diabetes, heart disease, hypertension, blood sugar intolerance, hyperlipidemia (especially elevated triglycerides and decreased HDL), polycystic ovary syndrome, elevated uric acid, refractory weight gain, fatty liver (steatosis), and calcium oxalate kidney stones. Often the individual with metabolic syndrome has a history of failing at numerous weight-loss diets, especially low-calorie, low-fat, high-carbohydrate diets. Discussion with the patient often includes comments regarding cravings for carbohydrates and starches, being "addicted" to sugar, falling asleep after meals, erratic energy, having headaches and being "grouchy," and awakening from sleep needing a snack during the night.

Besides obesity, people with metabolic syndrome often have a history of gestational diabetes, large babies, carbohydrate cravings, and abnormal liver enzymes associated with a fatty liver.

Physical examination may show apple-shaped obesity with an enlarged waist circumference (greater than 40 inches in men or 35 inches in females), dermatological findings like acanthosis nigricans (a dark pigmented rash under the arms, breasts, or back of the neck) and skin tags, ear lobe crease, arcus senilis (a white ring on the cornea), hirsutism (facial hair) in females, and elevated blood pressure. The two lists below summarize these features.

Past Medical History of Typical Metabolic Syndrome Patients

- non-European ancestry
- gestational diabetes
- borderline blood sugar levels
- resistant obesity
- gout
- sleep apnea
- elevated triglycerides, low HDL
- abnormal liver enzymes, fatty liver

- hypertension
- large babies
- hypoglycemia
- calcium oxalate stones
- carbohydrate cravings
- polycystic ovary syndrome
- low energy, sleepiness after eating

Physical Findings in Metabolic Syndrome

- elevated blood pressure
- acanthosis nigricans
- earlobe crease
- abdominal obesity (enlarged waist circumference) — 40+ inches in males and 35+ inches in females

- skin tags
- arcus senilis
- hirsutism

ıll Laboratory Findings for Metabolic Syndrome

Common laboratory findings in metabolic syndrome include elevated triglycerides, depressed HDL, a triglyceride/HDL ratio greater than 4.0, impaired blood sugar tolerance (fasting blood sugar from 100–126, hemoglobin A1C 6.0–6.5), fasting insulin greater than 8 and/or an elevated two-hour postprandial (after eating) insulin above 50. Metabolic syndrome researcher Dr. Gerald Reaven recently expressed his view that clinicians can make a diagnosis of metabolic syndrome without insulin levels. He advises clinicians to be more influenced by the presence of elevated triglycerides and low HDL cholesterol.[6] Insulin resistance correlates with elevated levels of cardiosensitive CRP-hs, a marker for cardiovascular inflammation. Elevated homocysteine levels are also associated with insulin resistance. Many patients with a fatty liver have nonspecific mild elevations of liver function tests. Other lab markers that have been reported include low magnesium and DHEA levels, and high serum ferritin and fibrinogen levels. Lab markers showing promise on the research level include adiponectin and interleukin-6. These factors are summarized in the list below.

Common Metabolic Syndrome Lab Findings

- elevated triglycerides, decreased HDL, triglyceride/HDL ratio in excess of 4.0
- borderline fasting blood sugar of 100–126
- two-hour postprandial (after eating) insulin 50+
- elevated C-reactive protein (cardiosensitive)
- mild, nonspecific elevations of liver function tests
- increased ferritin levels (iron storage)
- decreased serum magnesium
- fasting insulin greater than 8
- hemoglobin A1C 6.0–6.5
- elevated homocysteine
- elevated uric acid

- decreased DHEA levels
- hepatic steatosis (fatty liver)

ıl Treatment Options for Metabolic Syndrome

The following questions will introduce you to the central treatment concept of eating low-glycemic foods.

1. If you have metabolic syndrome, does it make any difference if you eat an 80-calorie piece of white bread or an 80-calorie piece of 100 percent whole-grain rye bread? After all, they are both bread and equal in calories.

2. If you have metabolic syndrome, does it make any difference if you eat an 80-calorie cookie or raw almonds totaling 80 calories? After all, they are both snacks, and they contain the same number of calories.

3. If you have metabolic syndrome, does it make any difference if you eat a 75-calorie apple or a 75-calorie banana? After all, they are both fruit and have good nutritional value.

The correct answer to each question is yes; it does make a difference. The best choices are the 100 percent whole-grain rye bread, the raw almonds, and the apple. In order to break the vicious cycle of excessive insulin production in response to high-glycemic foods, it is desirable to abort this cycle by consistently making choices to eat low-glycemic-index foods. In these examples, the successful patient with metabolic syndrome learns to consistently make the low-glycemic choice, rather than settle for the argument that all calories are equal, which implies the choices are equal. In my experience, for their particular genomics and metabolic status, metabolic syndrome patients feel better, lose weight more quickly and effectively, and normalize their blood pressure, blood sugar, and triglycerides more quickly with low-glycemic food plans.

As we discussed earlier, the glycemic index (GI) measures the effect of

> Metabolic syndrome patients feel better, lose weight more quickly and effectively, and normalize their physiology more quickly with low-glycemic food plans. Low-glycemic-index foods cause a lower glucose release, leading to a decreased insulin response.

a food on blood sugar. Indirectly, it also measures insulin response. The glycemic index ranks glucose at an arbitrary figure of 100. Foods with a GI over 55 have a moderate to high-glycemic-index. See Table 4.1 below for examples of glycemic index values. The key idea for metabolic syndrome patients is that low-glycemic-index foods cause a lowered glucose response and thus decreased insulin secretion.

Table 4.1: Examples of Foods and the Glycemic Index

LOW (BELOW 55)	INTERMEDIATE (55–70)	HIGH (70+)
Berries	Banana	Dried dates, raisins
Apples	Pineapple	Rice cakes
Cherries	Shredded Wheat, Special K	Corn flakes, most cereals
Barley	Oatmeal (cooked), brown rice	White rice
Bulgur	Whole-grain breads	Potatoes, white and red
Peanuts	Popcorn	White and wheat bread
Kidney beans, lentils	Pita bread, rye crackers	Pretzels, jellybeans
Green beans	Beets	Taco shells

ıl Not All Fat Is Bad

Healthy fats, if not eaten to excess, can be very helpful in the metabolic syndrome diet. Polyunsaturated fats found in corn, soybean, and safflower oil help lower LDL cholesterol. Monounsaturated fats, found in olive, canola, and peanut oil, also help lower LDL cholesterol. At the same time, they may protect LDL cholesterol from being oxidized, a dangerous process that encourages the buildup of plaque on artery walls and can lead to heart disease. Different types of fats can have different effects on glycemic response and insulin binding. A higher polyunsaturated/-saturated fat ratio improves cellular responsiveness to insulin. Taking fish oil supplements has been found not only to improve insulin sensitivity but also to prevent diabetes-induced nerve damage. The American Heart Association recommends fish oil supplementation for coronary disease prevention, especially in the presence of high triglycerides.[7]

Healthy fats, like monounsaturated fats and polyunsaturated fats, improve the glucose release and insulin response in patients with metabolic syndrome.

ıı Fiber Is Also Helpful

Fiber plays an important role in insulin and glucose response. High fiber intake, independent of total carbohydrates, has a positive effect on blood glucose control and cholesterol. Soluble fibers, in particular, act favorably on blood insulin concentrations. Examples are oat bran and psyllium powder. Fiber in the diet appears to slow gastric emptying, and to a lesser extent, inhibits starch degradation in the upper small intestine. In general, increasing the proportion of low-glycemic carbohydrates, healthy fat intake, and intake of soluble fiber usually improves the glycemic index of a meal or snack.[8]

> Soluble fiber improves glucose release and insulin response in patients with metabolic syndrome. Increasing the proportion of low-glycemic carbohydrates, and/or increasing healthy fat and soluble fiber, usually improves the glycemic index of a meal or snack.

In almost all metabolic syndrome patients, it is good to remember that when the patient is able to lose 5 to 10 percent of his or her fat mass, the vicious cycle of insulin resistance and hyperinsulinemia can be broken. Unfortunately, this can be exceedingly difficult to do, as the blood sugar/insulin abnormalities of metabolic syndrome vigorously defend themselves and are extremely resistant to traditional dietary interventions.

ıı Micronutrients Play a Role

Omega-3 fatty acids have a beneficial effect on plasma insulin and lipid concentrations. When these beneficial fatty acids are included in the diet of research subjects, insulin resistance in skeletal muscle is prevented. Good sources of omega-3 fatty acids include flaxseed or flaxseed oil, pumpkin seed, chia seeds, walnuts, almonds, and cold-water fish such as salmon. We frequently recommend 1 gram of EPA/-DHA twice daily as part of our metabolic syndrome treatment plan.

Research has confirmed a definite relationship between chromium and glucose tolerance. Recent studies have examined the use of chromium in type 2 diabetes and suggest that fasting and postprandial blood sugar (after eating) and insulin are significantly reduced with chromium supplementation. We usually start our metabolic syndrome patients on chromium 200 mcg twice daily.

At the cellular level, a number of other micronutrients may help support and stabilize the insulin signal and glucose utilization (see Table 4.2). These micronutrients include conjugated linoleic acid (CLA), lipoic acid, vanadium, magnesium, vitamin E, inositol, and biotin.

Table 4.2: Micronutrient Supplements to Help Relieve Metabolic Syndrome (Daily Intake)

SUPPLEMENT	DAILY INTAKE
Glucose tolerance factor chromium	100–600 mcg
Magnesium glycinate	100–400 mg
Vanadyl sulfate	100–500 mcg
Conjugated linoleic acid (CLA)	1,000–3,000 mg
Alpha lipoic acid (ALA)	100–500 mg
EPA/DHA	2–4 grams
Biotin	100–200 mcg
Inositol	500–1,000 mg
Vitamin E	100–400 iu

ıı Medications Have a Place

The vast majority of our metabolic syndrome patients are treated successfully without prescription medications. However, at times insulin sensitizers, fat-blocking, and anorectic medications can be used. I suggest that you consider them only after a detailed and careful discussion with your health practitioner about their relative risks and benefits. Sometimes, in difficult and relapsing cases, patients need to explore all options.

Insulin Sensitizers

Two currently available insulin sensitizers are metformin and thiazolidinedione drugs (TZDs). TZDs decrease insulin resistance in the tissue, including skeletal muscle and in the liver, resulting in increased insulin-dependent glucose disposal and decreased hepatic glucose output. Studies have shown no clinically significant drug interactions between TZDs and warfarin, digoxin, nifedipine, acarbose, metformin, glyburide, ranitidine, or fibrate therapy. Patients with active liver disease should not be started on TZDs. Patients taking TZDs should have a routine liver test every other month for the first year of therapy and periodically thereafter. Weight gain and fluid retention may be side effects associated with TZDs.

Metformin enhances the uptake of glucose into the muscle and lowers insulin levels about 20 percent. It is not associated with weight gain or hypoglycemia. If gastrointestinal side effects occur with metformin, they can be minimized with a low starting dosage. One important precaution applies to the use of this drug. Because it has to be cleared by the kidneys, patients with impaired renal function should not take this medication. This use of metformin for metabolic syndrome is considered "off-label" and may require written informed-patient consent.

Anorectic Agents

Since weight loss is the key to successful metabolic syndrome management, some patients might consider anorectic medications agents as part of a comprehensive approach. This approach ideally should include behavior modification, nutrition education, and increased physical exercise.

Orlistat blocks approximately 35 percent of ingested fat from absorption and allows it instead to pass out of the body mixed with the stool. Long-term studies have shown risk factor reduction in obese patients treated for two years with this drug. It does not interfere with the absorption of medications such as phenytoin, warfarin, digoxin, glyburide, nifedipine, or oral contraceptives. Because of its action, side effects—especially if a meal contains excess fat—include a loose, oily stool, oily flatulence, or oily seepage from the rectum. Since some fat-soluble vitamins like A, D, E, and K may be decreased with use of orlistat, a multivitamin should be taken daily.

Sibutramine works as an appetite suppressant. Its most common side effect has been the increase of blood pressure in some patients. Common, mild, transient side effects are headache, increased sweating, and an increase in heart rate.

Phentermine and its derivatives have been available for many years. The mechanisms of action may be on the appetite-control centers of the hypothalamus, but this has not been confirmed. It is contraindicated in patients with heart disease, uncontrolled hypertension, and narrow angle glaucoma. The most common side effect is dry mouth; to a lesser extent, feeling "hyper" and insomnia can also be problematic. Unlike orlistat and sibutramine, phentermine has never been approved for long-term use.

ıı A Nutriceutical Designed for Metabolic Syndrome

In addition to eating low-glycemic-index foods that include soluble fiber and healthy fats, we have been amazed at the results produced by utilizing a medical food designed for nutritional support of individuals with insulin resistance and hyperinsulinemia. UltaGlycemX is a powdered beverage mix formula that contains 15 grams of soy protein, 17 mg of soy isoflavones, and 9 grams of fiber per serving. It is free of dairy, lactose, wheat, gluten, egg, yeast, artificial colors, and artificial flavors. It does not contain stimulants, preservatives, artificial flavoring, or artificial coloring. Ingredients also include chromium, alpha-lipoic acid, vanadium, and magnesium, all of which have been shown to improve the body's regulation of glucose and insulin.

> A nutriceutical medical food specially designed for metabolic syndrome issues is Ultra-GlycemX, made by Metagenics Inc. (www.metagenics.com).

Perhaps the most important ingredient, however, is high-amylose starch, which, in contrast to typical starches in the diet, is broken down very slowly and released from the stomach into the bloodstream gradually after ingestion. This leads to a long, slow release of glucose, smoothing out the patient's blood sugar and insulin response. This unique proprietary blend, when combined with soluble fibers from guar and locust bean gum, slows the rate of gastric empty-ing and thus improves the glycemic response. My patients and I absolutely love this product and the results

> We use a medical food designed to normalize glucose and insulin levels. It is an integral part of the program, containing micronutrients, soluble fiber, and a unique, specially developed high-amylose starch (slow-release starch), which are very effective in helping our patients feel better, improve glucose and insulin levels, and lose weight.

it helps us to achieve. Moreover, patients are amazed at their ability to go several hours without hunger or blood sugar swings after using the product. As a result, this metabolic syndrome nutriceutical improves patients' overall sense of well-being, productivity, and ability to function. Sadie's story, which follows, is typical of how this medical food can be the key to remarkable weight loss and improvement in a patient with metabolic syndrome.

Sadie's Story

Controlling "Apple"-Shape Obesity

Sadie's lifelong history of obesity had greatly escalated after the births of her three children. By age 44, she had tried many programs for weight reduction but had encountered only frustration and failure. She had recently taken the prescription drug metformin for insulin resistance, but she could not tolerate it. Her medical history included polycystic ovary syndrome; irregular, prolonged menstrual cycles; and borderline blood sugars. Sadie's family history was positive for diabetes mellitus. Physical examination revealed the apple shape common to metabolic syndrome, hirsutism (unwanted facial hair), thinning of hair on the scalp, and skin tags.

Sadie's Initial Evaluation

Height: 5 feet, 6 inches
Weight: 343 pounds
Waist circumference: 51 inches
Blood pressure: 146/84 (nl: 130/80)
Body fat: 44.7 percent (nl: 25)
Fasting blood sugar: 100
Fasting insulin: 21.8 (nl: 8)

Recommendations

We recommended that Sadie initiate the following regimen:

1. Start a 1,200- to 1,400-calorie Cavewoman Diet. After losing 10 percent of original weight, continue with 1,200- to 1,400-calorie, low-glycemic-index food plan. Use metabolic syndrome medical food, two scoops each morning.

2. Start additional supplements of EPA/DHA 1 gram twice daily, and inositol 500 mg twice daily.
3. Commit to regular walking, at least 150 minutes per week.
4. Keep careful daily diet and exercise records.
5. Drink 64 ounces of water daily.
6. See Dr. Rigden and staff regularly for monitoring, education, and motivation.

2-Month Follow-Up
Sadie's weight is 307 pounds, and her blood pressure is 108/76. (Total weight loss: 36 pounds)

4-Month Follow-Up
Sadie's weight is 278.2 pounds, and her blood pressure is 118/76. (Total weight loss: 44.8 pounds)

6-Month Follow-Up
Sadie's weight is 256 pounds, and her blood pressure is 116/65, fasting blood sugar is 92. Fasting insulin is now 8.4. (Total weight loss: 67 pounds)

7-Month Follow-Up
Sadie's weight is 250.4 pounds, and her blood pressure is 102/68. (Total weight loss: 93 pounds)

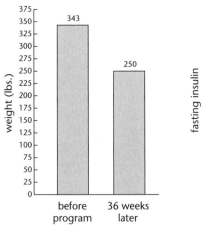
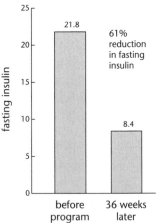

FIGURES 4.7 AND 4.8. Sadie's weight loss and insulin levels

Summary

	INITIAL	FINAL
Weight	343 pounds	250.4 pounds
Blood pressure	146/84	102/68
Fasting insulin	21.8	8.4
Fasting blood sugar	100	92

ııl Two Dietary Interventions

Two dietary interventions are needed in order to succeed in treating the switched metabolism associated with metabolic syndrome. The first intervention, which is a bit difficult but necessary and extremely effective to get your metabolism moving in the direction of fat burning, is the Caveman/Cavewoman Diet. After either losing the first 10 percent of your fat mass and/or reaching your weight loss goal, we then recommend you follow the FMRC low-glycemic-index diet, a healthy and effective approach, for the rest of your life!

> Two dietary interventions are needed to succeed with the switched metabolism associated with metabolic syndrome:
>
> 1. The Caveman/Cavewoman Diet "jump-starts" the process.
>
> 2. The FMRC low-glycemic-index diet maintains the weight loss for life.

Because obesity associated with switched metabolism and metabolic syndrome can be so difficult to break through, we have found the Caveman/Cavewoman approach an important and effective first step to kick-start your metabolism to burn fat and for you to lose weight. It is a healthy and extremely safe food plan to follow for weeks or months at a time, with a supplementary multivitamin-mineral tablet. Females should also consider taking supplemental calcium. Once they are on it, our patients positively embrace this diet because of its simplicity, and because they are thrilled with the results!

1. The Caveman/Cavewoman Diet Jump-Starts Weight Loss

Sample Menu

Breakfast	Medical food designed to help metabolic syndrome, two scoops each morning
Morning Snack	1 piece of low-glycemic fruit (equivalent servings include): ½ grapefruit, 15 cherries or grapes, 1 cup of berries, 1 medium orange or apple
Lunch	4 ounces nonfat cottage cheese *or* 3 ounces lean beef *or* 4 ounces fish, chicken, or turkey + 2 to 4 cups of salad greens with 1 tablespoon of equal parts vinegar and olive oil *or* 1 tablespoon of commercial olive oil-based dressings
Afternoon Snack	1 piece of low-glycemic fruit (see above)
Dinner	Protein: 4 ounces lean beef *or* 6 ounces fish, chicken. or turkey 2 to 4 cups of salad greens with dressings as noted above 1 to 2 cups of steamed nonstarchy vegetables
Evening Snack	3 ounces turkey, chicken, nonfat cottage cheese, *or* one hardboiled egg, with one low-glycemic fruit *or* one low-glycemic fruit, with 10 raw almonds
Any Time	Raw vegetables as munchies (see list below)

Raw Vegetables and Salad Fixings

- asparagus
- brussels sprouts
- celery
- green beans
- mushrooms
- radish
- watercress

- broccoli
- cabbage
- cucumber
- kale
- onions
- spinach
- tomato, fresh (1 small)

- zucchini
- cauliflower
- endive
- lettuce
- peppers

Condiments

- basil
- lemon

- cinnamon
- garlic

- dill
- mustard

- nonstick oil spray   ▪ oregano   ▪ parsley
- salsa (unsweetened)   ▪ pepper   ▪ vinegar

More Tips
- Drink at least eight 8-ounce glasses of water daily. In addition, you may have up to 16 ounces of decaf coffee, tea, or diet soda.
- Exercise daily, at least 20 minutes.
- Record food intake and exercise daily.
- Supplements:

   Multivitamin-Mineral: _____
   Calcium 500 mg/day: _____
   Other supplements as directed by your health adviser:

   _____

In Chapter 3, I introduced my colleague Barb Schiltz and asked her to share thoughts on the FMRC low-glycemic diet as a treatment program for carbohydrate sensitivity. As an expert on the clinical use and application of low-glycemic diet concepts for metabolic syndrome, she will now share more of her practical wisdom.

Tips for Dieters   by Barbara Schiltz

Does it feel as though you are always hungry? Does it seem like you are always thinking about food? Are you craving carbs in particular? It must be a relief to know that help is on the way! The higher the glycemic index of your diet, the more you will continue to crave foods high in carbohydrates. Each time you ingest a high-GI food your blood sugar will spike, causing a higher-than-optimal insulin response. Subsequently, this response will cause your blood sugar to plummet, leading you to eat again. We discussed this cycle previously, but it is critical for you to understand what is happening so you can make a shift. If you continue to choose high-GI foods, your eating habits will continue to be out of control. This vicious cycle will continue until you are able to make the necessary changes.

I suggest that my patients consider their first visit with me as "the beginning of the rest of your life." Imagine the power in this statement! What a life-altering thought this can be. This is not a diet per se, but a total lifestyle change that you are *choosing* because you wish to be healthier.

It is important to think more about the foods you are encouraged to eat, rather than to focus on feeling deprived. An abundance of delicious foods is available, but you must be willing to take the time to plan each meal rather than just "letting it happen." Red wine has recently been studied for its positive effect on cardiovascular disease. For this reason, we allow one or two glasses of red wine, three or four times per week, for our patients who already have been drinking wine. We do not encourage people who don't drink to start. It does have some benefit, however, and knowing you can have an occasional glass of wine might make this program feel more doable, particularly if you are someone who enjoys wine.

Look at the following menu plans. Many of the foods we suggest can also be eaten as leftovers in subsequent days. It always makes sense to prepare more than you need for one meal.

In Chapter 3 I presented the general principles of following the FMRC low-glycemic-index diet and listed all the foods by food groups. Here are two days of sample meals and menus that a person with metabolic syndrome might choose to follow. Also, there are a number of delicious low-glycemic recipes that I have developed, which are located in the Recipes section in the back of the book.

2. FMRC Low-Glycemic-Index Diet Maintains Weight Loss

Sample Menus: 1,800-Calorie Program

Day 1

Breakfast	Protein shake
Morning Snack	1 pear or apple and 8 walnut halves (*servings:* 1 fruit, 1 nuts)
Lunch	¾ cup black bean soup ½ sandwich: 3 ounce roast turkey breast on 1 slice 7-grain bread garnished with 1 teaspoon canola mayonnaise, lettuce, and sliced tomato 1 cup fresh blueberries ¾ cup nonfat or low-fat cottage cheese (*servings:* 1 legume, 1 grain, 2 proteins, 1 oil, 1 fruit)
Afternoon Snack	Protein shake and 15 cherries

(cont'd.)

Day 1 (cont'd.)

Dinner	3 ounces broiled salmon
	1 cup steamed spinach, topped with garlic sautéed in 1 teaspoon olive oil
	1 small baked sweet potato
	Salad:
	  1–2 cups mixed greens
	  ⅓ cup green soy beans
	  ¼ cup each raw broccoli and cauliflower
	  ½ stalk diced celery
	  ½ medium tomato
	  8 green olives
	  ⅛ avocado
	  1 tablespoon oil and vinegar dressing
	  (*servings:* 1 protein, 1 legume, 5 oil, 1 category 2 vegetable, free veggies)

Evening Snack	Vegetable salsa dip:
	  ⅓ cup salsa, comprised of the following:
	    1 whole cucumber
	    ½ cup each raw green beans
	    sliced red pepper
	  (*serving:* free veggies)

Total: 1,800 calories (45 percent carbohydrate, 27 percent protein, 28 percent fat, 57 grams dietary fiber)

Day 2

This could be a weekend day, when you want to have a real, cooked breakfast.

Breakfast	Vegetable omelet:
	  2 whole eggs or 1 whole egg and 3 whites
	  ¼ cup chopped spinach
	  2 tablespoons sliced mushrooms
	  Spray pan with olive oil spray before cooking (or coat with ¼ teaspoon oil). Sauté mushrooms first, then add eggs.
	½ cantaloupe cut into wedges
	(*servings:* 1 protein, 1 fruit, free veggies)

Morning Snack	Protein shake

(cont'd.)

Day 2 (cont'd.)

Lunch	Large tossed salad: 2 cups shredded mixed greens 3 ounces either leftover or canned chunk lite tuna ½ cup each garbanzo or kidney beans raw broccoli cauliflower ¼ cup cucumber slices ½ medium tomato ¼ avocado, cut into chunks Toss with 1 tablespoon vinegar and oil dressing. 3 Ryvita crackers with 1 tablespoon almond butter 1 medium peach or 1 whole grapefruit (*servings:* 1 protein, 1 legume, 1 grain, 1 nut, 1 fruit, free veggies, 4 oil)
Afternoon Snack	Protein shake
Dinner	¾ cup split pea, lentil, or black bean soup Chicken vegetable stir-fry: 3 ounce chicken breast, cut into strips, stir-fried in 1 teaspoon olive oil (remove chicken from pan before stir-frying the veggies) Stir-fry 1 carrot, sliced, ½ cup pea pods, ½ cup each red or green pepper strips and sliced onion, and 1 clove minced garlic in 1 teaspoon olive oil with 1–2 teaspoons fresh minced ginger. Add stir-fried chicken, soy sauce, salt, and pepper to taste. 1 cup baked spaghetti squash, topped with above stir-fry (*servings:* 1 protein, 1 legume, 1 category 2 vegetable, free veggies, 2 oil)
Evening Snack	1 cup raspberries topped with 6 ounces plain nonfat or low-fat yogurt (*servings:* 1 dairy, 1 fruit)

Total: 1,800 calories (46 percent carbohydrate, 25 percent protein, 29 percent fat, 58 grams dietary fiber)

Harry's Story

At age 46, Harry had been experiencing progressive weight gain for the past 10 year. His blood pressure and blood sugar levels were borderline. He underwent a cardiac ablation procedure for an arrhythmia (abnormal rhythm). He tended to gain his weight in the "apple" configuration and had a positive family history for diabetes mellitus.

Harry's Initial Evaluation

Height: 5 feet, 10 inches
Weight: 262.4 pounds
Blood pressure: 140/88 (nl: 130/80)
Waist circumference: 45.5 inches
Body fat: 29.5 percent
Cholesterol: 171
Triglycerides: 69
HDL: 48
LDL: 112 (nl: 10)
Fasting blood sugar: 107 (nl: 100)
Fasting insulin: 8

Recommendations

We recommended that Harry initiate the following regimen:

1. Start the Caveman Diet of 1,200 to 1,400 calories, with a medical food designed for metabolic syndrome, two scoops each morning. After losing 10 percent of original weight, continue with a 1,200- to 1,400-calorie, low-glycemic-index diet plan.
2. Keep careful daily records.
3. Commit to regular visits to physician for monitoring, education, and motivation.
4. Exercise a minimum of 150 minutes a week.
5. Take supplements, including chromium 200 mcg twice daily, lipoic acid 200 mg twice daily, and EPA/DHA 1 gram twice daily.

1-Month Follow-Up

Harry's weight is 242 pounds, and his blood pressure is 120/70, fasting insulin 6.3, fasting blood sugar 90. (Total weight loss: 20.2 pounds)

3-Month Follow-Up

Harry's weight is 226.8 pounds, and his blood pressure is 118/62. (Total weight loss: 35.7 pounds)

6-Month Follow-Up

Harry's weight is 222.4 pounds, his blood pressure is 102/60, his waist circumference is 40 inches, and his percent body fat is 23.4. (Total weight loss: 40.1 pounds)

8-Month Follow-Up
Harry's weight is 212.2 pounds, and his blood pressure is 102/72. Harry's waist circumference is 38 inches. He has lost 50.2 pounds.

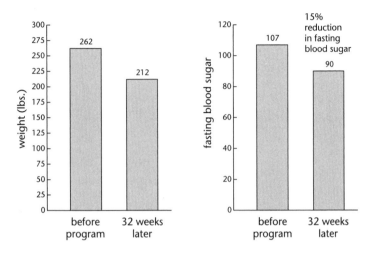

FIGURES 4.9 AND 4.10. Harry's weight loss and fasting blood sugar results

Summary

	INITIAL	FINAL
Weight	262.4 pounds	212.2 pounds
Waist circumference	45.5 inches	38 inches
Blood pressure	140/88	102/72
Body fat	29.5 percent	23.4 percent

Helen's Story

By age 48, Helen had been dealing with weight problems since her youth. She had a medical history that included giving birth to a large baby (9 pounds, 6 ounces), hirsutism (facial hair), and gestational diabetes. Her family history was positive for heart disease, stroke, and hypertension. She was on thyroid replacement medication. She tended to gain weight in the "apple" distribution.

Helen's Initial Evaluation
Height: 5 feet, 7 inches
Weight: 268.2 pounds
Blood pressure: 118/70
Waist circumference: 48.5 inches
Body fat: 48.2 percent
Fasting blood sugar: 88
Fasting insulin: 9.5 (nl: 8)
Two-hour postprandial (after eating) blood sugar: 117
Two-hour postprandial (after eating) insulin: 84 (nl: 25)

Recommendations
We recommended that Helen initiate the following regimen:

1. Start the Cavewoman Diet of 1,200 to 1,400 calories, with a medical food designed for metabolic syndrome, two scoops each morning. After losing 10 percent of original weight, continue with a 1,200- to 1,400-calorie, low-glycemic-index diet plan.
2. Initiate chromium 200 mcg twice daily, lipoic acid 200 mg daily, and EPA/DHA 1 gram twice daily.
3. Exercise at least 150 minutes per week.
4. Keep careful daily records.
5. Commit to regular physician visits for patient education, motivation, and monitoring.
6. Drink at least 64 ounces of water daily.

2-Month Follow-Up
Helen's weight is 250.6 pounds, and her blood pressure is 116/70. (Total weight loss: 17.6 pounds)

4-Month Follow-Up
Helen's weight is 237.8 pounds, and her blood pressure is 118/70. (Total weight loss: 30.4 pounds)

6-Month Follow-Up
Helen's weight is 229.4 pounds, and her blood pressure is 102/60, fasting insulin 4.2, two-hour postprandial (after eating) insulin 16. (Total weight loss: 39.2 pounds)

9-Month Follow-Up
Helen's weight is 217.6 pounds, her percent body fat is 32.0, and her waist circumference is 43 inches

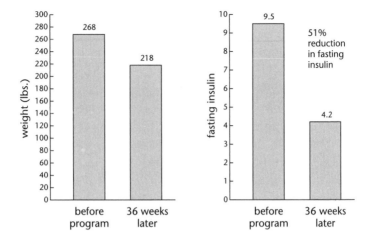

FIGURES 4.11 AND 4.12. Helen's weight loss and insulin

Summary

	INITIAL	FINAL
Weight	268.2 pounds	217.6 pounds
Waist circumference	48.5 inches	43 inches
Body fat	48.2 percent	32 percent
Insulin	9.5	4.2

Laura's Story

Laura, at age 50, had been gaining weight steadily in the six years since her hysterectomy, which led to estrogen replacement therapy (ERT). She also had suffered from extreme fatigue for the past two years, stating that her low energy and malaise felt like having a case of mononucleosis. She rated her energy below 50 percent of her normal level. Her family history was positive for diabetes mellitus type 2.

Laura's Initial Evaluation
Height: 5 feet, 5 inches
Weight: 173.2 pounds
Blood pressure: 118/72

Fasting insulin: 11.4 (nl: 8)
Fasting blood sugar: 109 (nl: 100)
Cholesterol: 247 (nl: 180)
HDL: 73
LDL: 143 (nl: 130)
Triglycerides: 157 (nl: 150)

Initial Program Recommendations
We recommended that Laura begin the following program:

1. Start the Cavewoman Diet of 1,200 to 1,400 calories. After losing 10 percent of original weight, continue with a 1,200- to 1,400-calorie, low-glycemic-index diet plan.
2. Take two scoops of a medical food designed for metabolic syndrome each morning, along with twice-daily supplements of chromium 200 mcg, lipoic acid 200mg, and EPA/DHA 1 gram.
3. Keep careful daily food records.
4. Commit to regular physician visits for monitoring, patient education, and motivation.
5. Drink at least 64 ounces of water daily.
6. Exercise a minimum of 150 minutes weekly.

6-Week Follow-Up
Laura's weight is 158.2 pounds, with blood pressure at 115/76. (Total weight loss: 15 pounds)

10-Week Follow-Up
Laura's weight is 154.6 pounds, with blood pressure at 118/72. (Total weight loss: 18.6 pounds)

14-Week Follow-Up
Laura's weight is 151.6 pounds, with blood pressure at 118/78. (Total weight loss: 21 pounds)

18-Week Follow-Up
Laura's weight is 144.7 pounds, and her blood pressure is 106/68; lab results include fasting blood sugar 85, cholesterol 171, HDL 60, LDL 96, and triglycerides 77. (Total weight loss: 27.9 pounds)

28-Week Follow-Up
Laura's weight is 141.8 pounds. The patient has excellent energy and is exercising daily. (Total weight loss: 30.8 pounds)

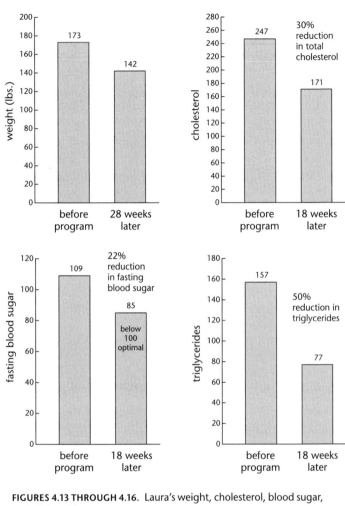

FIGURES 4.13 THROUGH 4.16. Laura's weight, cholesterol, blood sugar, and triglycerides

Summary

	INITIAL	FINAL
Weight	173.2 pounds	141.8 pounds
Blood pressure	118/72	106/68
Cholesterol	247	171
Triglycerides	157	77
HDL	73	60
LDL	143	96

The case studies in Chapters 3 and 4 involve the two most common causes of switched metabolism, carb sensitivity and metabolic syndrome. The reader should know these case studies reflect typical results of patients in our office on the programs discussed in these chapters. I have randomly reviewed the records of 32 patients who in 2005 had either carb sensitivity or metabolic syndrome. They were on my programs from 12 to 52 weeks and lost between 12.6 to 108 pounds, with an average weight loss of 35.6 pounds.

Hormonal Imbalances

ıl Hormonal Imbalances Screening Questionnaire

Part A: For Men and Women

Circle the number of any statement that applies to you.

1. My family history is positive for thyroid problems.
2. I frequently feel cold when others are comfortable.
3. My face and body are often puffy or swollen.
4. I am very sluggish in the morning and have difficulty in getting up.
5. My hair appears to be unhealthy or is falling out.
6. My skin has become overly dry.
7. My nails are brittle.
8. I have a history of high cholesterol.
9. I am taking Synthroid or another thyroid replacement.
10. I have significant issues with decreased libido.
11. My weight gain has coincided with very high stress.
12. I have gained weight distributed in my upper back below the neck level.

Part B: For Women Only

1. I experience food cravings and weight gain with PMS.
2. My weight gain has been associated with perimenopause or menopause.
3. My weight gain has been associated with taking hormone replacement therapy or the birth control pill.
4. I have abnormal menstrual cycles.
5. I have had difficulty getting pregnant.
6. I have had ovarian cysts, documented either by ultrasound and/or laparoscopy.
7. My menstrual cycles usually are very uncomfortable/painful.
8. Unwanted facial hair has become a problem.
9. I have had thinning of the hair on the top of my head.
10. I have had a tendency to have acne and/or seborrhea (dandruff).
11. I have continued to gain weight even though I have tried to reduce.
12. I tend to carry my body fat in the "apple" distribution.
13. I have skin tags around my neck and upper body.
14. I have been told my blood sugar is abnormal or borderline.
15. I have had to take birth control pills or have had surgery for gynecological symptoms.

Answer Key: If you circled five or more statements in part A, your lifestyle and genomics have probably combined to create hormonal abnormalities, which are a major factor in perpetuating your weight problem and keeping you from success in a weight-loss program. If you have circled two or more statements from questions 1–3 in Part B, it is likely that you have estrogen dominance, a type of hormonal imbalance that contributes to switched metabolism. If you have circled five or more statements from questions 4–15 in Part B, you likely have polycystic ovary syndrome (PCOS).

ııl Glossary of Medical Terms Used in Chapter 5

adrenal glands: These glands are located on the kidneys. They are first-line responders to stress and release large amounts of cortisol and adrenaline-like hormones in response to stress.

ACTH (adrenocorticotropic hormone): This is an adrenocorticotropic hormone that is released by the pituitary and stimulates the adrenal gland to release more cortisol, a key stress hormone.

adaptogenic medicinal plants: These are plants such as Panax ginseng, Siberian ginseng, Rhodiola crenulata, and Cordyceps sinensis that contain herbs that may enhance the body's anti-stress defense mechanisms.

alopecia: Hair loss.

amenorrhea: Lack of menses.

CRH: Corticotropin-releasing hormone is released by the hypothalamus in response to stress; this hormone stimulates the pituitary to release ACTH.

cruciferous vegetables: These cabbage family vegetables include broccoli, Brussels sprouts, cabbage, cauliflower, bok choy, collards, kale, kohlrabi, mustard greens, radish, rutabaga, turnip, and watercress.

DHEA: Dihydroepiandrosterone is an important hormone secreted by the adrenal gland; it is often abnormal in PCOS patients.

estrogen: The main female hormone secreted by females; typically there are three kinds of estrogen: estradiol, estrone, and estriol.

HRT: Stands for hormone replacement therapy, used for perimenopausal or menopausal females; this can be done with pharmaceuticals or natural bio-identical hormones.

indole-3-carbinol: Nutrient found in cruciferous vegetables that influence estrogen metabolism.

infertility: The inability to conceive.

LH/FSH: Hormones released by the pituitary gland that are often abnormal in PCOS patients. LH stands for luteinizing hormone and FSH stands for follicle-stimulating hormone.

menopause/perimenopause: Menopause refers to total cessation of menstrual cycles in the female; perimenopause refers to the period of time between normal menstrual cycles and menopause, often defined by irregular menses, spotting, and/or heavy menstrual flow.

phytoestrogens: Naturally occurring plant nutrients that cause mild estrogen-like activity in the body; examples are isoflavones in soy and lignans in flaxseed.

PMS: Premenstrual syndrome. Symptoms are weight gain, bloating, and irritability that occur in susceptible females three to seven days prior to menses.

polycystic ovary syndrome (PCOS): This condition affects 6 to 10 percent of women of reproductive age. It is the most common cause of anovulatory infertility, in which females have menstrual cycles without ovulation. Seventy percent of PCOS women are obese. Elevated levels of androgen, ovulation problems, and ovarian cysts define this condition.

progesterone: A female hormone secreted when ovulation occurs.

Synthroid: A common prescription of T4 (thyroxine).

testosterone: The main androgenic hormone in females; it is often abnormally high in females with PCOS.

T4, T3: The thyroid gland releases T4 (thyroxine), which circulates in the bloodstream and attaches to receptors in many organs of the body. Some of the body's T4 is transformed to T3 in the liver; T3 is very important for burning fat.

thyroid gland: A gland located at the base of the neck that is a key player in weight loss metabolism and the production of physical energy.

TSH: Stands for thyroid stimulating hormone, which is released from the pituitary to stimulate the thyroid to release thyroid hormone; it is also measured in the most commonly measured lab test to determine if the thyroid is over or underactive.

ιιι Thyroid Hormone Imbalances

The leading unrecognized hormonal imbalance that I see is in the area of thyroid abnormalities. This fact is not surprising when experts at the University of Colorado Medical School have recently reported that the prevalence of mild thyroid failure occurs in approximately 10 percent of the general population and in up to 20 percent of older women. Richard Shames, MD, in his book *Thyroid Power*, notes, "By age 60, one woman out of every six is hypothyroid."[1]

Dr. Shames also notes the following:

- You could have low thyroid despite a normal TSH test.
- You could still be low thyroid despite any normal thyroid test.
- The above two situations may occur regardless of whether you are being diagnosed for the first time or are being checked after years of treatment.
- If your blood tests are normal, but you haven't been tested for thyroid antibodies, insist on this as a next step. Even more sensitive than TSH and antibody determination is the TRH test.
- More important, the greatest test of all is how you feel—rather than a laboratory number.

Even with normal TSH (thyroid-stimulating hormone) screening tests, a troubling number of my overweight patients have continued to have thyroid-related symptoms. In addition, even with thyroid treatment, they continued to have classic symptoms of an underactive or sluggish thyroid (hypothyroidism). These symptoms included low body temperature, cold extremities, dry skin, adult acne or eczema, mild depression, dry hair, hair loss, and fatigue. In addition, common complaints may be morning sluggishness, brittle nails that crack or peel easily, menstrual irregularity, and carpal tunnel problems. It is also common for these people to have a positive family history of thyroid problems, high cholesterol, and autoimmune disorders.

Frequent physical findings of a sluggish thyroid may include listlessness, thick tongue, prominent bags under the eyes, abnormal size or shape of the thyroid gland, and difficulty swallowing. The skin is often dry or rough, body temperature may be below normal, and water retention may be present. Also, a physician should look for slow pulse, low blood pressure, and thinning scalp hair.

Hypothyroid patients have physical symptoms that may have previously been ignored. These symptoms can include listlessness, thick tongue, prominent bags under the eyes, abnormal shape or size of the thyroid gland, and difficulty swallowing. These patients may also have skin that is dry or rough, low body temperature, water retention, slow pulse, low blood pressure, and thinning scalp hair. A subtle clinical indication is the loss or thinning of the outer one-third of the eyebrows.

ıl Why the Diagnosis Is Missed

Primary care physicians often fail to recognize sluggish thyroid because of their early medical training. In a nutshell, we doctors were taught that if the basic thyroid panel and TSH are normal, the patient has normal thyroid function. Period. End of discussion! Although my opinion is still considered controversial, I maintain that a mildly low-thyroid individual can still appear normal on paper. Overweight patients often have a sluggish metabolism even with a normal TSH test. According to our clinical experience, as well as the experience of experts like Dr. Richard Shames, a TSH over 3.0 is considered suspicious, and anything over 4.0 merits treatment, particularly if accompanied by other signs, symptoms, or family history. Even when the normal limits in the lab are 0.4–5.4, we aim for control in the 0.5–2.5 range.

Almost all thyroid hormone in the bloodstream is tightly bound to blood carrier protein. In this form, it is not available to enter the cells. A small fraction, however, is free and ready to enter the cells immediately. It is possible to measure the small fraction of free T3 and free T4.

The common assumption that if a person has a normal TSH and T4 level, he or she must also have a normal level of circulating T3 is not always warranted. When the system is working in perfect balance, about 5 percent of circulating T4 is converted to T3 by enzymatic reactions in the liver. However, the efficiency of this system can by compromised by variables such as imbalances of adrenal and sex hormones, environmental toxins, auto-immune reactions, and poor

> If you have doubts about whether your thyroid status is normal, consider a free T3 test.

nutrition. Approximately 20 percent of our overweight patients with switched metabolism have low free T3 counts.

Josie's story illustrates how a metabolic problem caused by failure to convert T4 (thyroxine) efficiently to T3 in the body can result in switched metabolism and weight gain along with other troubling symptoms. This baffling case was resolved by giving the patient a small amount of T3 and encouraging the adoption of the Mediterranean diet.

Josie's Story

Thyroid Mystery

At age 47, Josie came to our office with complaints of an extremely difficult weight problem. She was also experiencing low energy, memory loss, irritability, and depression. She had been evaluated at a prestigious medical institution in the Southwest and had been told to see a psychiatrist. She tried several antidepressants, which did not help any of her symptoms. In addition, she had seen numerous other practitioners to no avail. Regarding the weight, she had gained 35 pounds over the past two years and had tried several rigorous dieting efforts to lose the weight with no results. She also suffered from dry skin, swelling of the hands and feet, and hair loss. Extensive lab work had been within normal limits.

Josie's Initial Evaluation

Height: 5 feet, 5 inches
Weight: 185 pounds
Josie's TSH thyroid test was normal, but her Free T3 count, which had not been checked by multiple practitioners, was low-normal at 2.5 (the limits of normal being 2.3–4.2).

Recommendations

Josie started a supplement of T3, 25 mcg daily, and immediately started feeling increased energy, relief of the hair loss and dry skin, and improved energy. In addition, she started to lose weight by consuming a modified Mediterranean diet. In eighteen months she had reduced her weight to 158 pounds, and in two years she weighed 148 pounds. She has continued to feel great, is off all medications except the T3, and has maintained her weight for four additional years.

ıl Dr. Rigden's Favorite Protocol

My favorite thyroid protocol for patients with a suspicious clinical history, normal or borderline TSH, and a low free T3 is as follows. Start with time-released T3, formulated by a clinical pharmacist, 7.5 mcg each morning. Gradually increase the time-released T3, according to lab and clinical response, up to 12.5 mcg twice daily.

The reader may be taking thyroid replacement such as Synthroid or Levothyroxine, which contains only thyroxine (T4). Nevertheless, if the TSH lab test is within normal limits but greater than 3 and you have symptoms of hypothyroidism, consider asking your doctor about obtaining a free T3 count. If the T3 count is depressed, you may want to add T3 to your T4 supplement, or consider switching to a different thyroid medication that contains both T4 and T3.

> If you are already taking thyroxine (T4), it may be helpful to add T3 to your regimen or to switch to a form of thyroid containing T4 and T3.

ıl Problems of Estrogen Dominance

Estrogen dominance may lead to any of the following:

- weight gain
- fibrocystic breasts
- uterine hyperplasia
- borderline hypothyroidism
- PMS
- fibroids
- water retention

Estrogen-dominant women often experience food cravings and weight gain with PMS. They may also report large weight gain while going through menopause or perimenopause. With these women, weight gain is often associated with taking hormone replacement therapy or the birth control pill. In addition to clinical suspicion, estrogen dominance can be confirmed with serum or salivary hormone level testing.

> Estrogen dominance is caused by a relative excess of estrogen in relation to progesterone. These women often experience food cravings and weight gain with PMS. They may also report large weight gain while going through menopause or perimenopause. Weight gain is often associated with taking hormone replacement therapy or the birth control pill.

Many overweight women with switched metabolism have estrogen dominance—that is, a relative excess of estrogen in relation to progesterone. During the menstrual cycle, some of these women may not produce enough progesterone to balance their estrogen production. In other cases, they may have suboptimal metabolism and detoxification of estrogen. This, in turn, leads to a buildup of a form of estradiol that causes symptoms of estrogen dominance. To simplify a very complicated subject, the main form of estrogen in the body, estradiol, may be metabolized in the liver through Phase I (hydroxylation) and Phase II (methylation, glucuronidation, and sulfation) pathways. The three possible fates of estradiol metabolism are the 2-OH metabolite, the 4-OH metabolite, and the 16-aOH metabolite. The 2-OH metabolite causes very weak estrogenic activity and is generally termed the "good estrogen." The metabolites in the 4-OH and 16-aOH pathways tend to cause the symptoms of estrogen dominance. In addition to weight issues, these "bad estrogens" confer increased risk for uterine and breast cancer.

Beneficial modulation of estrogen metabolism can be accomplished through dietary and lifestyle modifications, such as increasing fiber intake, reducing dietary fat intake, and increasing one's intake of phytoestrogens (e.g., isoflavones in soy, lignans in flaxseed, and certain flavonoids in citrus fruits and grapes). Losing weight, increasing exercise, and increasing one's intake of certain nutrients may also help this process. These nutrients include indole-3-carbinol, found in cruciferous (cabbage family) vegetables, B vitamins, magnesium, limonene, and antioxidants such as lipoic acid, vitamin C, and vitamin E. Cruciferous vegetables include bok choy (Chinese cabbage), broccoli, Brussels sprouts, cabbage, cauliflower, collards, kale, kohlrabi, mustard greens, radish, rutabaga, turnip and turnip greens, and watercress.

ıl Treatment Strategy for Estrogen Dominance

If you have estrogen dominance and are on hormone replacement therapy (HRT), with the approval and knowledge of your doctor consider discontinuing standard pharmaceutical hormone therapies like Premarin and Estrace. Then, working with your physician and a compounding pharmacist, substitute bioidentical natural progesterone, topical or oral. This strategy lowers estrogen dominance and leads to improved weight loss. Always consult your healthcare practitioner before initiating a new hormone supplementation program.

> Estrogen-dominant women can benefit from taking bioidentical natural progesterone, topical or oral.

In addition, lifestyle modifications implementing the strategies listed above that can cause preferential metabolism of estradiol to the "good" 2-OH pathway are helpful. Our basic estrogen modification program consists of a daily high-quality soy protein drink for the isoflavones, a diet employing moderate amounts of healthy fats, moderate exercise, one heaping teaspoon of flaxseed meal daily, 800 mcg of folic acid daily, and a serving of cruciferous vegetables daily for indole-3-carbinol.

> Estrogen-dominant women can benefit from daily intake of a high-quality soy protein drink for isoflavones, a diet containing moderate amounts of healthy fats, moderate exercise, flaxseed meal, folic acid, and cruciferous vegetables (for indole-3-carbinol).

ıl Polycystic Ovary Syndrome (PCOS)

This syndrome affects 6 to 10 percent of women of reproductive age. It is the most common cause of anovulatory infertility (having a menstrual cycle without ovulation). Seventy percent of women with PCOS are obese. The definition of PCOS includes elevated levels of the male hormone testosterone, ovulation problems, and ovarian cysts (usually documented on ultrasound).

> PCOS is defined by elevated levels of testosterone, ovulation problems, and ovarian cysts.

Hirsutism (in this case, the presence of unwanted facial hair) affects 70 percent of PCOS women. Their fat distribution is in the "apple" shape. They often have thinning hair on the top of the head and acne and/or seborrhea. In addition, they may exhibit skin tags around their neck and upper body, acanthosis nigricans (a dark pigmented rash), and a waist circumference often exceeding 35 inches.

PCOS affects 6 to 10 percent of women of reproductive age. It is the most common cause of infertility in this group. Seventy percent of PCOS women are obese. Elevated levels of androgen, ovulation problems, and ovarian cysts define PCOS.

The lab results of PCOS women often show decreased sex hormone binding globulin (SHBG), elevated free or total testosterone, LH/FSH ratio greater than 3, elevated DHEA, and elevated insulin levels or evidence of insulin resistance. They often have borderline or abnormal blood sugar readings, abnormal blood sugar tolerance tests, and abnormal hemoglobin A1C tests (that measure long-term blood sugar levels).

Table 5.1: Testing for PCOS

TESTS FOR PCOS	TYPICAL PCOS RESULT
Sex hormone binding globlin (SHBG)	Decreased
Androstenedione	Increased
Free testosterone	Increased
Total testosterone	Increased
DHEA	Increased
Fasting insulin	8+
Fasting blood sugar	100–126
LH/FSH	Greater than 3
Triglyceride/HDL ratio	Greater than 4

ıl The Goals of PCOS Treatment

The primary goal of treatment is to reduce or normalize insulin resistance. This enables the body to reduce elevated androgens, improve endometrial (uterine) function, enhance fertility, attain a healthier weight, and improve appearance. Normalizing insulin status leads to a remarkable chain of events that helps the body to normalize the other associated hormonal imbalances. We have found that a weight-management program with a low-glycemic-index diet; an exercise program; a specially designed soy protein powder with slow-release high-amylose starch to facilitate the attainment of normal blood sugar and insulin levels (such as UltraGlycemX, made by Metagenics Inc.); and supplements including chromium 200–400 mcg daily, inositol, 500–600 mg twice daily, EPA/DHA 1–2 grams twice daily, and lipoic acid 200 mg twice daily is very effective.

> The key components of PCOS treatment are a low-glycemic-index diet, an exercise program, the use of a specially designed soy protein powder with slow-release high-amylose starch to facilitate attainment of normal blood sugar and insulin levels, and the use of supplements including chromium, inositol, EPA/-DHA, and lipoic acid.

Nadia's story illustrates the treatment principles noted above and happily ends with successful weight loss and a pregnancy after years of infertility.

Nadia's Story

Overcoming PCOS
At age 27, Nadia had a 10-year history of confirmed PCOS with erratic, long, painful menses, and she was experiencing thinning hair. She had intermittently been on contraceptive pills for this period of time. Without them, she had a menstrual cycle only every six months. She had a positive pelvic ultrasound confirming the presence of polycystic ovaries and had tried using metformin, with no benefit, for about six months. She had been gaining weight steadily over the past ten years in the "apple" configuration. Her family history was positive for cancer and stroke.

Nadia's Initial Evaluation
Height: 5 feet, 5 inches
Weight: 222.2 pounds
Blood pressure: 146/90
Waist circumference: 38 inches
Body fat: 34.3 percent

Cholesterol: : 206 (nl: 180)
Triglycerides: 217 (nl: 150)
HDL: 37 (nl: 50)
LDL: 126
TSH: 2.18
Fasting blood sugar: 95
Fasting insulin: 31 (nl: 8)

Nadia's prolactin, FSH (follicle-stimulating hormone), LH (luteinizing hormone), and fasting cortisol, frequently abnormal in cases of PCOS, were all within normal limits; however, her testosterone levels were all abnormally increased.

Assessment

We determined that Nadia was suffering from the following conditions:

1. PCOS
2. hypertension
3. obesity
4. insulin resistance
5. hyperlipidemia
6. abnormal testosterone levels
7. infertility, amenorrhea (lack of menses), and alopecia (hair loss) associated with PCOS

Recommendations

We recommended that Nadia begin following the following program guidelines:

1. Start 1,200- to 1300-calorie low-glycemic-index food plan, using a specially designed soy protein powder with slow-release, high-amylose starch to facilitate attainment of normal blood sugar and insulin levels, two scoops each morning.
2. Commit to regular physician visits for patient education, motivation, and monitoring.
3. Walk at least 30 minutes daily.
4. Keep careful daily records.
5. Initiate chromium picolinate 200 mcg twice a day, EPA/DHA 1 gram twice a day, lipoic acid 200 mg twice a day, and inositol 600 mg twice daily.

1-Month Follow-Up
Nadia's weight is 201.8, and her blood pressure is 127/86. She is experiencing normal menses after 3 months of amenorrhea. (Total weight loss: 20.4 pounds)

3-Month Follow-Up
Nadia's weight is 184.6, and her blood pressure is 118/70. She is experiencing normal menses. (Total weight loss: 35.6 pounds)

4-Month Follow-Up
Nadia's weight is 177.2 pounds. Her blood pressure is 112/65, percent body fat: 28.1. Nadia's waist circumference is 32.25 in. She is experiencing normal menses. (Total weight loss: 45 pounds)

5-Month Follow-Up
Nadia's weight is 173.4 pounds. Her blood pressure is 102/60, cholesterol 190, triglycerides 55; HDL, 46; LDL, 133. Her fasting is insulin 7.3 and her free testosterone is 1.8, both of which are normal. She is experiencing normal menses. She feels great and is starting to have fuller, thicker hair. (Total weight loss: 48.9 pounds)

7-Month Follow-Up
Nadia's weight is 170.6 pounds. Her blood pressure: is 106/64, waist circumference is 32 inches, percent body fat is 29.0. She is experiencing normal menses. (Total weight loss: 51.6 pounds)

8-Month Follow-Up
Nadia's weight is 172.0 pounds. Her blood pressure is 102/62. Nadia has lost 50 pounds, is feeling great, and is pregnant!

17-Month Follow-Up
Patient delivers a healthy baby!

Summary

	INITIAL	5 MONTHS
Weight	222 pounds	173 pounds
Blood pressure	146/90	102/62
Fasting insulin	14.2	7.3 (normal)
Waist	38	32 (measured at 7 months)

(cont'd.)

Summary *(cont'd.)*

	INITIAL	5 MONTHS
Triglycerides	217	55
Free testosterone	4.7	1.8
Menses	amenorrhea	normal
Head hair	thin	normal

ɪɪl The Cortisol-Stress Connection

Dr. Hans Selye won the Nobel Prize for his work on the role of stress and the adrenal glands in understanding health and human physiology. Dr. Selye defined the general adrenal adaptation syndrome, which states that given any source of external biological stress, an organism will respond with consistent biological patterns of adaptation in an attempt to restore its internal homeostasis. In its most basic form, the stress response involves this chain of events: a person has to adjust to altered environmental circumstances; the hypothalamus releases more corticotrophin-releasing hormone (CRH); in response to the increased CRH, the pituitary releases more adrenocorticotropic hormone (ACTH), which stimulates the adrenal gland to release more cortisol, a hormone that helps the body deal with stress.

Among its many benefits, cortisol helps us fight inflammation and allergies, maintains blood pressure and blood sugar, balances electrolytes, and helps maintain a strong immune system. Concurrently with the above steps, the sympathetic nervous system is activated with an alarm response that stimulates the release of catecholamines, like adrenaline, to mobilize the body for a "fight-or-flight" response.

ɪɪl Phases of Adrenal Response to Stress

Dr. Selye explains that there are three phases of adrenal response to chronic stress. Phase One, the adaptation phase, involves intermittent slightly higher levels of adrenal hormones in response to a slightly higher level of stress. Phase Two, the alarm phase, occurs when consistent high stress causes excessive levels of adrenal hormones to be released. Phase Three, the exhaustion phase, involves atrophy of the adrenal glands, which then put out insufficient levels of hormone. During the alarm phase, under the influence of unrelenting high levels of cortisol, many of our patients gain extraordinary amounts of weight.

> During the alarm phase of the adrenal response to high stress levels, some patients gain extraordinary amounts of weight under the influence of unrelenting high levels of cortisol.

ıl Understanding Stress and Weight Gain

Robert Sapolsky, PhD, a noted stress researcher from Stanford University, has defined stress physiology as the reaction of the body "to imperfections in our world and the attempts of our bodies to muddle through them." [2] These circumstances frequently occur in our complicated modern lifestyles and can include extreme stress from challenges in a personal, professional, family, or health area. When I ask many of my obese patients to gauge their perception of stress in their lives on a scale of 0–10 during a time of rapid weight gain, they often report they are "off the scale with a level of 10 plus." It is no wonder some people can produce very high levels of cortisol that are comparable to those of an individual who has had to take high levels of cortisone-based medication for a long period of time or who has contracted Cushing's Syndrome, an adrenal gland medical condition of overproduction of cortisol. Similar to the individual who has had to take prednisone in high doses for a prolonged period of time, some overweight patients' bodies will exhibit rapid weight gain, fluid retention, upper-body obesity, rounded or "moon" facial appearance, and a fat pad just below the neck in the upper mid-back called a "buffalo hump." In addition, the resemblance between the Phase Two alarm adrenal response-related weight gain, Cushing's, and the associated use of steroid medication, also often includes elevated blood sugar, insulin resistance, and high blood pressure.

> High levels of cortisol produced during stress can cause rapid weight gain, fluid retention, upper-body obesity, rounded facial appearance, and fat deposits below the neck in the upper back. Increased blood sugar, insulin resistance, and high blood pressure can also result.

Moreover, high levels of ACTH and cortisol can alter the conversion of T4 to T3. Often our obese patients who have been under chronic high stress need extra T3 support. The trend in medicine seems to be moving toward salivary testing of the adrenals for evaluation of cortisol levels. Taking four separate samples of saliva is frequently more revealing, giving the physician a better chance to evaluate circadian rhythm. It is also more convenient than a blood draw at the lab.

ııl Stress Reduction Lowers Cortisol-Related Weight Gain

Stress reduction is the key to controlling this problem. You are encouraged to work with a professional with whom you have a good rapport and who is experienced in stress management. This could be a physician, psychologist, counselor, or pastor. With objective professional help, you can achieve more adapt ability and flexibility in your personal and professional life. Relationships and self-esteem can be improved with hard work and persistence. Effective counseling can supply the skills, tools, information, and support through which you can make healthy changes.

Stress-Management Exercise

1. Take three slow breaths, emphasizing a long exhalation.

2. Count slowly to 10.

3. Repeat, "I am a calm, confident, peaceful, poised person."

Exercise, meditation, biofeedback, and yoga are helpful for many of our patients. Sometimes a simple stress-management strategy that includes some of the following suggestions can be used to help improve a difficult day.

Helpful lifestyle changes may include acquiring a pet, cultivating a new hobby or outside interest, improving time management, controlling your telephone and schedule more effectively, modifying your physical work environment, developing inspiration and humor files, improving sleep quality, and decreasing or eliminating the use of alcohol, caffeine, and tobacco.

Other beneficial lifestyle changes may include acquiring a pet, cultivating a new hobby or outside interest, working with a time-management consultant, controlling your telephone time and managing your schedule more effectively, modifying your physical work environment, developing inspiration and humor files you can consult and use regularly, improving sleep quality, and decreasing or eliminating the use of alcohol, caffeine, and tobacco.

ıl Nutritional Support for the Adrenal Glands

Nutritional support for the overused and abused adrenal gland includes the inclusion of vitamin C 1,000 mg daily, B-complex 50 mg three times daily, and pantothenic acid 500 mg daily. If you are working with a health professional who is well versed in adaptogenic medicinal plants, ask about including a dosage of Panax ginseng, Siberian ginseng, Rhodiola crenulata, and Cordyceps sinensis. Although their use is controversial in mainstream medicine, an increasing number of reports suggest these compounds may positively enhance the body's antistress defense mechanisms.

Food Hypersensitivities

ııl Food Hypersensitivity Screening Questionnaire

Circle the numbers of any statements that apply to you.

1. As an infant or small child I had problems with colic, allergies, or recurrent respiratory infections.
2. I have a past or current medical history of asthma.
3. I have a past or current medical history of chronic nasal or sinus problems.
4. I have a past or current medical history of hives or eczema.
5. I have a past or current medical history of irritable bowel syndrome.
6. I have a past or current medical history of excessive headaches.
7. I have a past or current medical history of musculoskeletal aches and pains.
8. I eat wheat or milk-based foods several times a day.

Answer Key: If you have circled three items, it is possible that food hypersensitivities are contributing to your weight problem. If you have circled four or more items, it is likely you have significant food hypersensitivities that are contributing to your weight problem and switched metabolism.

142

ıll Glossary of Medical Terms Used in Chapter 6

asthma: An allergic disorder marked by difficulty in breathing, wheezing, and a cough.

eczema: An itching skin rash marked by oozing and then crusted lesions.

elimination diet: A diet that omits certain foods for 30 to 90 days that trigger food hypersensitivity reactions. The foods omitted can be those identified by RAST testing or they can be part of a standardized diet that is discussed in Chapter 6.

food hypersensitivity: An abnormal reaction of the immune system to certain trigger foods in the diet. This reaction involves excessive release of antibodies from the immune system that are usually provoked by microbes or pollens. These reactions can cause the release of toxins that can cause symptoms such headaches, skin rash, aches and pains, congestion, stomach problems, fluid retention and weight gain.

IgE antibodies (immunoglobulins): Proteins usually released by the immune system to protect the body from allergens such as pollen or insect stings.

IgG antibodies (immunoglobulins): Proteins usually released by the immune system to protect the body from microbes.

inflammatory cytokines: Disruptive, toxic chemicals that cause swelling, pain, redness, or itching. In the context of this chapter, they can be released in response to a reaction of IgG antibodies to food breakdown particles in the bloodstream.

irritable bowel syndrome: A disorder of the colon that is characterized by abnormal elimination patterns; these can be marked by loose, urgent, frequent stools, diarrhea, gas, bloating, and constipation. Sometimes there is alternating diarrhea and constipation.

RAST test: A blood test that is able to detect increased levels of IgG and/or IgE antibodies that the body has released in response to a trigger food.

ıll The Physician's Perspective

I strongly suspect food hypersensitivity when a patient has issues with switched metabolism and also has a strong history of allergies throughout his or her life. Although the patient's physical examination may be completely normal, there are sometimes subtle, physical findings. These may include allergic shiners (dark circles under or around the eyes), mouth breathing, boggy or swollen nasal mucosa, wheezing, eczema, and hives. Frequently, these individuals appear listless, lethargic, and sleepy. They often complain of fluid retention and swelling in the extremities, sometimes literally gaining two pounds of fluid weight overnight!

> Overweight patients with food hypersensitivities often have a strong history of lifelong allergic tendencies. Their physical exam often demonstrates allergic shiners, mouth breathing, swollen nasal membranes, wheezing, eczema, and hives.

Melanie's Story

Melanie was age 29 when she came to our office for help. In spite of vigorously dieting and working out at the gym with a personal trainer, Melanie simply could not lose weight. In addition, she had a long-standing history of allergies, asthma, and eczema, and she felt very sluggish. She had numerous laboratory tests from various physicians that were within normal limits. Her initial measurements included height of 5 feet 3 inches and weight of 176.6 pounds. Her physical examination revealed allergic "shiners," swollen nasal membranes compatible with allergy, skin rashes on her hands and around the scalp, and wheezing in the lungs. A RAST test for food hypersensitivities showed extremely high reactions to corn and wheat. As a result, we started Melanie on our modified elimination diet, with special emphasis on completely eliminating corn and wheat. She was encouraged to continue to exercise regularly. Twelve weeks later she weighed 157.2 pounds (a loss of 19.4 pounds). Moreover, her skin was almost clear, her nasal and lung symptoms had markedly improved, and she had 50 percent more energy.

Sherry's Story

Sherry came to our office following many years of frustration. By age 35 she had failed in repeated attempts to lose weight, In addition, her energy on a typical day was only 60 percent of normal. A history of a thyroid condition, called Hashimoto's thyroiditis, may have contributed to her weight problem; however, this had been treated by a specialist for eight years and was said to be under good control. At one time she was found to have had a mildly elevated insulin level and was treated with the prescription drug, metformin, but to no avail. More recently, she had undergone two knee surgeries, which had temporarily limited her exercise program. Extensive laboratory testing at our office showed excellent results, except for results to her RAST test for food hypersensitivity. Sherry had very strong reactions to multiple foods, including wheat, dairy, soy, eggs, beef, lamb, almonds, and all beans. Laura received extensive dietary counseling on how to implement an elimination diet that omitted her reactive foods. To ensure enough protein in her diet, she also was started on a hypoallergenic, rice-based protein powder, two to four scoops daily. Laura was encouraged to continue her aerobic exercise regime of 45 minutes daily and to drink 64 ounces of water daily. Twenty weeks later her weight was 135.2 pounds (a loss of 41.2 pounds) and she had outstanding energy. When she comes into the office, she calls her program "my miracle diet."

ıll How Food Hypersensitivities Cause Weight Gain

Three mechanisms may help explain how food reactions cause weight gain. These are: (1) release of excessive water into the cells to dilute and lessen the impact of toxic inflammatory chemicals; (2) inflammatory chemicals released by food/IgG antibody complexes can interrupt fat metabolism; (3) exorphins (addiction-prone chemical substances released from partially digested foods) cause craving and overeating of trigger foods.

The first mechanism involves food hypersensitivity reactions that cause the release of excessive water into the cells to dilute and lessen the impact of toxic inflammatory chemicals. In other words, "the body's solution to pollution is dilution." *Pollution* in this case refers to toxic chemicals (inflammatory cytokines) released into the bloodstream as the result of an adverse reaction to a specific food. Your immune system,

> Food hypersensitivities may cause weight gain by triggering release of excessive water into the cells to dilute and lessen the impact of toxic inflammatory chemicals.

metaphorically speaking, has an infantry that fights foreign invaders and wants to protect you from microbes, insect stings, reactive foods, and so forth. Some foods can disagree with your body and disrupt its healthy chemistry in an instant and violent way, such as eating peanuts and immediately having your throat swell. This potentially life-threatening reaction is caused by "foot soldiers" in your immune system who want to protect you. They belong to a group of protective antibodies called IgE immunoglobulins. In this case, the IgE type of antibody group can dangerously overreact to an allergic food.

But in the case of switched metabolism and food hypersensitivities, we are talking about a delayed immune system reaction that is subtle and may not manifest for 24 to 72 hours after the offending food has been consumed. For example, eating wheat on Monday and feeling tired and achy on Tuesday with a significant weight gain is typical for our patients with switched metabolism and food hypersensitivities. This lower grade, smoldering immune-system reaction turns off fat metabolism and is caused by a different regiment of soldiers in your bloodstream; these "soldiers" are called the IgG immunoglobulin family. It is as if your IgG immunoglobulin "soldiers" try to protect you by reacting to the reactive foods, or "foreign invaders." This skirmish between your IgG immunoglobulins and the molecules of your reactive foods releases toxic chemicals. Called inflammatory cytokines by scientists, these toxic chemicals cause injury to your cells in the form of swelling and inflammation. These toxic chemicals build up in the tissues, triggering the body's cellular defense mechanisms to dilute or "water down" the pollutants to protect the cell and diminish the impact of the toxins. Many similar cellular reactions over weeks and months can multiply and readily explain the marked tendency toward water retention and fluid weight gain in many patients.

Second, inflammatory chemicals released by the food/IgG antibody interaction can interrupt fat metabolism. These toxins (scientists call them members of the prostaglandin E2 family that trigger inflammation in the body) may build up in the body as a result of repeated daily exposure and reactions and directly impact your fat cells. They are triggered by the interaction of your immune system's protective "soldiers," the IgG antibodies, with the "foreign invader," or reactive food. These toxins can powerfully disrupt your normal fat metabolism physiology and inhibit fat breakdown (lipolysis).

The third mechanism involves exorphins, addiction-prone chemical substances released from partially digested foods; these cause cravings for and overeating of trigger foods. This relatively new information helps explain the well-known clinical observation that "what you are allergic to, you are addicted to." This observation seemed paradoxical until biochemists clarified the exorphin theory. Exorphins are the opposite of endorphins. It is well known that endorphins are released after exercise, and help us to feel positive, happy, and productive. Exorphins, on the other hand, are released by addictive drugs and biochemical imbalances in the brain. They can make us feel negative, unhappy, and possibly depressed. Exorphins can be released by a siege in your bloodstream between the "good guys" (your IgG protective antibodies) and the "bad guys," (reactive foods); this conflict releases breakdown products from partially digested reactive foods. Exorphins, in other words, are toxic chemicals that can circulate to the brain and bind to certain areas of the brain that trigger "addiction" behavior, which can lead to craving for and overeating of reactive foods.

Food hypersensitivities cause weight gain through three mechanisms:

1. The body releases excessive water into the cells to dilute and lessen the impact of toxic inflammatory chemicals.

2. Inflammatory chemicals released by the food/IgG antibody interaction can interrupt fat metabolism.

3. Exorphins, addiction-prone chemical substances released from partially digested foods, cause craving for and overeating of trigger foods.

ıll Seeing the Picture Clearly

To review: In contrast to IgE-mediated food allergies, such as eating strawberries and immediately breaking out with hives, IgG-mediated food hypersensitivities cause chronic, ongoing symptoms. They often involve many foods and may be involved with chronic gastrointestinal problems like leaky gut syndrome (see Chapter 7). IgG-

> IgG-mediated food hypersensitivities can cause chronic, ongoing symptoms. IgG-mediated food hypersensitivities often involve many foods, may be associated with GI problems, and have a delayed onset, sometimes 24 to 72 hours after eating the food. Avoidance may be curative.

mediated food hypersensitivities have a delayed onset (sometimes 24 to 72 hours after ingestion of the food), and often may be "cured" by avoidance. The mechanism that causes symptoms is the deposit of toxins from the bloodstream into tissues—for example, the skin, gut, joints, or respiratory tract. These toxins result from a battle between your protective immune system "soldiers," the IgG antibodies, and the reactive foods. The diagnosis can often be confirmed with specific IgG blood tests, such as the RAST blood test.

ıl What Is the RAST Test?

The RAST test can diagnose your problem 93 percent of the time, according to Vincent Marinkovich, MD, a well-known specialist in the field of food allergies. Essentially, the RAST blood test involves very technical, new lab processes whereby extremely small quantities of a particular food are injected into a small drop of your body's blood. If you are nonreactive to this food, your immune system does not make antibodies (IgG immunoglobulins, the body's foot soldiers that try to protect you from foreign invaders). There is no observed, measurable clumping of your antibodies to the microscopic food particle. On the other hand, if you have a strong reactivity to a food, your immune system will release large numbers of IgG antibodies that will "attack" the food and cause a buildup of molecules that clump together and can be measured and quantified. The latter phenomenon would be a positive confirmation of a food hypersensitivity. Therefore, the test requires a blood specimen that is sent to the lab, where it is tested for reactions involving the most common 95 foods in the American diet.

ıl Treatment Options for Food Hypersensitivities

After a review of the RAST test for positive reactions, the patient is counseled on the necessity of strictly eliminating these foods for 90 days. Although 90 days may seem like a long time, the good news is that this interval usually is extremely effective in allowing you to re-introduce the offending foods after 90 days without the previous metabolic compromise. I repeat, *you do not have to avoid these foods forever!* An alternative to using the RAST test may be to employ a modified elimination diet to uncover possible reactive foods. This 90-day period of time is not arbitrary and is based on the following scientific observations. Over the first 30 days of abstinence, the high antibody levels will come down steadily because the immune system is not being regularly provoked. During the second 30-day interval (days 30 through 60), the patient feels significant relief from allergic symptoms and significant progress with weight loss. The third 30 day interval (days 60 through 90) enables the memory component of the immune system to "reset" so that it will, in most cases, be able to accept modest amounts of the previously offending food, especially if it is not eaten daily as before.

Food reactions can occur with any food. However, the most common problem foods are milk, wheat, and eggs. Because they are such staples of the American diet, abstinence from these foods is very challenging. I have asked my colleague nutritionist Barb Schiltz to share some advice she uses in counseling people on how to succeed with this daunting task.

Tips on Eliminating Wheat, Milk, and Eggs   by Barbara Schiltz

Helping patients avoid allergic foods is one of the most challenging issues in my clinical practice. Because we are most often allergic or sensitive to the foods we eat daily and crave, avoiding these foods typically requires a major change in daily food intake patterns. There is a period of withdrawal that usually lasts three or four days, during which you may experience mild to intense cravings for the addictive foods, along with a worsening of any chronic complaints you may currently have (headaches, joint aches, bloating, fatigue, and so on). Once you have passed this period, you may begin to experience a sense of well-being. During this period, many people report improvement in symptoms of brain fog, fluid retention, low energy, bloating and other digestive complaints, muscle and joint aches, and headaches. Weight loss begins to become apparent. It is truly worth the wait!

If you suspect or have been told you are allergic to dairy, wheat, and/or eggs, the following paragraphs will give you some practical advice.

Wheat is probably the most difficult food to eliminate. Many people have wheat toast, a muffin, and/or cereal for breakfast, a sandwich for lunch, and pasta or bread at dinner. Most desserts also contain wheat. What can you eat instead? A wonderful cookbook with recipes that omit wheat is *Gluten-free, Sugar-free Cooking* by Sue O'Brien.[1] (You will find sample recipes in the Recipes section at the back of this book, including one of my favorites, Sue's gingerbread.)

Bread is the most problematic food for which to find a substitute. Many wheat-allergic individuals don't care much for rice breads. When I counsel patients, I find it simpler to suggest totally avoiding breads because of their negative effects on blood sugar. Bread is usually the culprit that induces food cravings anyway. An occasional meal with a small amount of rice pasta can be quite tasty. My favorite brand of rice pasta is Tinkyada, found in most health-food stores. Rice crackers and rye crackers may also be acceptable bread substitutes, but you must be careful not to overeat these foods, because they may stimulate an exaggerated blood sugar response. Wheat-free cereals are available, and oatmeal is a satisfying hot breakfast food. Quinoa, a grain from South America, is available in flake form and can be used as a cooked cereal, and whole-grain quinoa has many uses. If you have a computer and are Internet-competent, you can find a number of recipes online by using Google or searching such sites as Epicurious.com.

Overall, when you are trying to lose weight, it is best not to eat too many grains, as most grains, except barley, tend to be high glycemic index (GI). Turkey breakfast sausage and a tofu scramble, with or without a low-glycemic soy shake, provide a filling breakfast. Legumes also contain carbohydrates but are very low in GI and thus help you feel satisfied after eating. Eating black bean salad or soup, lentil soup, hummus, chili made with kidney beans and ground turkey, or green salad with peas and/or garbanzo beans added is an easy way to incorporate low-GI legumes into your diet. Combining the low GI-grain barley with lentils or kidney beans and veggies in a soup or stew is a favorite with my patients.

Avoiding dairy can also be daunting, as common breakfast foods usually include some form of dairy: cottage cheese, yogurt, and milk added to cereal or coffee. Instead, rice, soy, or almond milk can be used on cereal or in coffee and tea, but they may take some getting used to. Cheese is also a frequent part of lunch and dinner. Unfortunately, most people don't care much for soy cheese and soy yogurt. Eggs are not quite as difficult to avoid, but eliminating them can limit choices even further, especially at breakfast, as eggs are typically viewed as good "diet food."

While you are on an elimination diet, eating at home is usually the path of least resistance, but if you are careful, you can also eat out in restaurants and have a pleasant meal. When dining in a restaurant, you have to become a detective, as wheat, milk, and eggs are often hidden ingredients in prepared foods. Did you know, for example, that soy sauce contains wheat? A wheat-free version, called "wheat-free tamari," is available in health-food stores. Tamari is a type of soy sauce that contains less salt. Not all tamari is wheat-free, however, so read the label carefully. Most restaurants do not use tamari, so some of my patients discreetly bring their own.

Breakfast is the most difficult meal to eat out when you are avoiding dairy, wheat, and eggs. Although these foods can be difficult to avoid in restaurants, I have found that most restaurant personnel are very cooperative when you inform them that you have specific food allergies. They can be helpful in suggesting alternatives. They want your repeat business, and they do not wish to incur any liability.

Oatmeal (moistened with fruit juice or applesauce) and fresh fruit are easy breakfast items to order in a restaurant, but you may find it easier to have a dairy-free protein shake at home and save dining out for lunch and dinner meals. Bean and veggie soups, green salads with fish or chicken, and entrees featuring broiled fish, chicken, or a lean steak, with vegetables and brown rice, are possible restaurant choices that all avoid dairy, wheat, and eggs. To avoid temptation, it might be wise to ask that your waiter not put bread on your table.

Uncovering food allergies or sensitivities are an important part of your program. Once you eliminate the offending foods, you allow your body to respond more efficiently to the rest of your program. With the removal of this roadblock, healing and weight loss can finally happen.

ıı The Next Step after 90 Days of Elimination

After 90 days of avoiding the suspect foods that tested positive on your RAST test, it is time to reintroduce them into the diet. The protocol is as follows:

Protocol for Reintroduction of Hypersensitive Foods

1. Eat two to three servings of the offending food in one day. Be careful not to introduce more than one food at a time. For example, if you are testing wheat, you could eat a serving with each meal, such as toast with breakfast, crackers with lunch, and pasta with your evening meal.

2. Observe your body carefully for the next 48 to 72 hours. Do you notice weight gain or fluid retention? Do you experience symptoms involving your upper respiratory tract, skin, or gut, or do you experience headaches? Do you have brain fog or fatigue? Do you have joint or muscle pain?

3. If you experience symptoms after you reintroduce the food, do not reinstate the food at this time. Instead, continue with another 30 days of abstinence before testing it again.

4. If you have no symptoms after introducing the food, reincorporate the food into the diet. You should have one serving of the food no more than one to three times a week, but not on consecutive days.

ıı A Modified Elimination Diet

As stated before, our modified elimination diet can be used as an effective diagnostic strategy for patients as an alternative to the RAST test. Patients whose allergic symptoms improve or clear while they are on the diet for 21 to 30 days have confirmed that food hypersensitivities are a significant area of health challenge; moreover, they usually also have impressive weight loss. After this period of elimination, the patient can systematically reintroduce suspected trigger foods according to the protocol discussed in the previous section on the 90-day elimination diet. In essence, the modified elimination diet is a safe and cost-effective diagnostic method of evaluating adverse reactions to foods in overweight patients. It also can be an effective therapeutic tool in achieving better health and weight loss.

The modified elimination diet developed by Barb Schiltz and her colleagues at the Functional Medicine Research Center in Gig Harbor, Washington, avoids most of the common food hypersensitivity culprits in our culture (see Table 6.1 on the next page)

Primary Guidelines

1. Eliminate all dairy products, including milk, cream, cheese, cottage cheese, yogurt, butter, ice cream, and frozen yogurt. Avoid products made with casein (a milk protein), such as soy cheese.

2. Eliminate fatty meats like beef, pork, and veal. Chicken, turkey, lean cuts of lamb, and cold-water fish such as salmon, mackerel, and halibut are acceptable if you are not allergic to or intolerant of these foods. Select free-range products whenever possible.

3. Eliminate gluten. Avoid any foods that contain wheat, spelt, kamut, rye, barley, or malt. This is the most difficult part of the diet, but it is also the most important. Unfortunately, gluten is in many common foods, including bread, cereal, pasta, crackers, and products containing flour made from these grains. Most individuals can safely select products made from rice, quinoa, millet, buckwheat, teff, and gluten-free flour, or potato, tapioca, or arrowroot.

4. Drink at least 2 quarts of water, preferably filtered water, daily.

5. Avoid all alcohol-containing products, including beer, wine, liquor, and over-the-counter products that contain alcohol. Also avoid all soda pop and other caffeine-containing beverages, including coffee and caffeine-containing tea. You should also avoid coffee substitutes made from gluten-containing grains, along with decaffeinated coffee. Be sure to read the labels of cold remedies and herbal preparations, as they frequently contain caffeine and/or alcohol.

Table 6.1: Modified Elimination Diet

FOOD GROUP	ALLOWED	AVOID
Meat, Fish, Poultry	Chicken, turkey, lamb Cold water fish such as salmon, halibut, mackerel, and trout	Red meat, cold cuts, frankfurters, sausage, canned meat
Legumes	All legumes, dried peas, lentils	Soy substitutes
Eggs	Cholesterol-free egg replacer (made from potato starch or flax seeds)	
Dairy Products	Milk substitutes such as rice milk, nut milks	Milk, cheese, cottage cheese, yogurt, ice cream, cream, non-dairy creamers, soy milk

(cont'd.)

Table 6.1: Modified Elimination Diet (cont'd.)

FOOD GROUP	ALLOWED	AVOID
Starch	White or sweet potato, arrowroot, rice, tapioca, buckwheat, millet, gluten-free products	All gluten-containing products, including pasta, all corn, and corn-containing products
Bread/Cereal	Any made from rice, quinoa, amaranth, buckwheat, teff, millet, potato flour, tapioca, arrowroot, or gluten-free flour-based products	All made from wheat, oat, corn, pelt, kamut, rye, barley, gluten-containing grains, corn-containing products
Vegetables	All vegetables, preferably fresh, frozen, or freshly juiced	Creamed vegetables or those made with prohibited ingredients
Fruits	Fresh, unsweetened, frozen, freshly juiced, or water-packed, canned fruits, excluding oranges	Fruit drinks, ades, cocktails, citrus, strawberries, and dried fruits preserved with sulfites
Soup	Clear, vegetable-based broth, homemade vegetarian soup, made with ground chicken or turkey, bean soup	Canned or creamed soup any with glutenous flours or chili grains
Beverages	Freshly prepared or unsweetened fruit or vegetable juice, pure water, non-citrus herbal tea, diluted fruit juices	Milk, dairy-based products, coffee, tea, cocoa, Postum, alcoholic beverages, soda pop, sweetened beverages, citrus drinks
Fats/Oils	Cold pressed, unrefined, light-shielded canola, flax, olive, grapeseed, pumpkin, sesame, and walnut oil, salad dressings made from allowed ingredients	Margarine, shortening butter, refined oils, salad dressings, and spreads
Nuts/Seeds	Almonds, cashews, flax seeds, pecans, pumpkin seeds, sesame, squash seeds, sunflower seeds, walnuts, nut/seed butters, pistachios	Peanuts and peanut butter
Sweeteners	Brown rice syrup, fruit sweeteners, agave nectar, honey, Stevia	Brown and white sugar, evaporated cane juice, maple syrup, corn syrup, molasses

ıı The Next Step after a 30-Day Modified Elimination Diet

The procedure uses the same protocol previously discussed after the 90-day elimination diet. To review, eat two to three servings of the offending food in one day. Be careful not to introduce more than one food at a time. Observe your body carefully for the next 48 to 72 hours. Do you notice weight gain or fluid retention? Do you experience symptoms involving your upper respiratory tract, skin, or gut, or do you experience headaches? Do you have brain fog or fatigue? Do you have joint of muscle pain? If you experience symptoms after you introduce the food, do not reinstate the food at this time. Instead, continue with another 30 days of abstinence before testing it again. If you have no symptoms after introducing the food, reincorporate the food into the diet. You should have one serving of the food no more than one to three times week, but not on consecutive days.

A common mistake when reinstating specific foods after a modified elimination diet is to consume combination foods, such as pizza, which contain both dairy and wheat. If you react to a combination food, you will not know which part of the food—for example, dairy or wheat—is causing the symptom. Instead of a combination food, use a food that is relatively pure. For example, a simple wheat challenge is a wheat tortilla for breakfast and/or lunch and plain pasta with sauce and/or vegetables for dinner. For a dairy challenge, milk and cheese are good choices, but ice cream is not because it also contains sugars. Proceed in this fashion with all the foods on the "avoid" list, keeping a careful record of any reactions. If you are not sure of a reaction, challenge the food again in the same way.

Another common problem I see is a lack of attention to refined sugars. My patients who have begun to feel better after a three-week, modified elimination diet sometimes tell me they had no reaction to any food that they reintroduced, yet when they go back on their usual diet, they slowly began to feel poorly again. This is because they have incorporated sugars back into their usual daily diet. Small amounts of sugar were initially okay, but larger amounts consumed on a daily basis appeared to have a cumulative, negative effect. Time and again, with reluctance and sometimes serious reservations, patients have told me that when they *finally* removed all refined sugars from their diet, all sorts of wonderful things happened. They had no more insomnia, fewer gastrointestinal complaints (especially heartburn and reflux), fewer food cravings, improved ability to lose weight, and an improvement in general mood or sense of well-being.

Did I say this was an easy task? I did *not*! Sweet foods are very addictive and no one finds eliminating them to be easy. Did I say it was worth a try? Yes!

ıl A Word about Artificial Sweeteners

It may be challenging to remove artificial sweeteners from your diet, because they are so universally accepted. However, the bottom line is that as long as you continue to drink diet sodas and eat other artificially sweetened foods on a regular basis, you will never really stop craving and thinking about sweet foods. Patients who have been unwilling to stop these so-called diet foods have never felt the relief from cravings for and obsessive thoughts about their favorite foods. Those who have weaned themselves off diet drinks happily admit what a relief it is to be consuming more healthy foods.

Ursula's Story

When she came to our office, Ursula had an extensive medical history of severe allergies, eczema, asthma, folliculitis (an infected skin rash involving the hair follicles), and dry skin since birth, in addition to being overweight. She also had battled hypoglycemia for many years. Allergy work-ups showed numerous inhalant allergies, which required monthly allergy injections. She knew she had food allergies to soy and peanuts, and she was allergic to penicillin. Ursula had tried to lose weight many times, including following commercial weight-loss programs, self-directed regimens, and working with a personal trainer, but with no success. At the time of this appointment she was working out with weights three times a week for a total of 120 minutes, combined with a rigidly disciplined 1,400-calorie diet, and she had not been able to lose weight. Medications included Estrace 0.5 mg daily. She had had a total hysterectomy and tonsillectomy in the past.

Physical Examination

Ursula's examination was very positive for allergic nasal mucosa, allergic shiners around the eyes, mild wheezing bilaterally, and eczema on the hands, forearms, and posterior scalp. Extensive dermatitis and folliculitis were noted on the face and legs.

Ursula's Initial Evaluation

Height: 5 feet, 5 inches

Weight: 179.2 pounds

Blood pressure: 168/71 (nl: 130/80)

Waist circumference: 37 inches

Hip circumference: : 45 inches

Cholesterol: 264 (nl: 180)

LDL: 154 (nl: 130)

Basic blood counts, TSH, liver function tests were all within normal limits.

Assessment

Ursula suffered from the following conditions:

1. obesity with associated inhalant and food allergies. Strongly suspect IgG-mediated food hypersensitivities
2. elevated systolic blood pressure
3. elevated cholesterol and LDL
4. allergic dermatitis, eczema, allergic rhinitis, and asthma
5. history of hypoglycemia

Recommendations

We recommended that Ursula initiate the following steps:

1. While waiting for RAST test results, initiate a 1,300- to 1,400-calorie, high-protein, low-carbohydrate diet, with five to six small meals per day. Every morning, have two scoops of a hypo-allergenic rice-based protein powder. (The hypoallergenic, rice-based protein powder Ursula used was UltraClear-Plus, made by Metagenics Inc. [www.metagenics.com].)
2. Check RAST test.
3. Keep careful daily records.
4. Continue weight training, with 20-minute walks four days per week.

5. Drink at least 64 ounces of water daily.
6. Commit to regular physician visits for monitoring, education, and motivation.

1-Month Follow-Up
Ursula's weight is 173 pounds. Her blood pressure is 164/90. Her RAST IgG results show very high reactions to 11 foods including egg, milk, corn, wheat, etc. Ursula starts an elimination diet. (Total weight loss: 6.2 pounds)

3-Month Follow-Up
Ursula's weight is 159.5 pounds. Her blood pressure is 143/89. Ursula's skin rashes and nasal and bronchial symptoms are much improved. (Total weight loss: 19.7 pounds)

5-Month Follow-Up
Ursula's weight is 150.4 pounds. Her blood pressure is 141/81. Her waist circumference is 33.5 inches, and her hip circumference is 39.25 inches. (Total weight loss: 28.8 pounds)

8-Month Follow-Up
Ursula's weight is 145.5 pounds. Her blood pressure is 145/93. Ursula's allergic rhinitis, asthma, and allergic skin conditions are all asymptomatic. The patient feels great. Her cholesterol is 202; her LDL is 110. (Total weight loss: 33.7 pounds)

Summary
Ursula implemented an elimination diet based on specific RAST testing, with further tailoring to her individual needs, consuming six small meals a day to control hypoglycemia and using supplementation with a hypoallergenic, rice-based protein powder. In eight months she was able to lose 33.7 pounds, improve her systolic blood pressure by 23 points, improve her cholesterol by 62 points and her LDL by 44 points, and lose a significant number of inches from her waist and hips. Moreover, her long-standing severe allergies were in remission.

Summary

	INITIAL	FINAL
Weight	179.2 pounds	145.5 pounds
Blood pressure	168/71	145/93
Cholesterol	264	202
LDL	154	110

■||||||||||||||||||||||||||||■

I find it interesting that most highly trained allergists still do not accept this theory as valid. So many people could potentially be helped by embracing what we now know in this area.

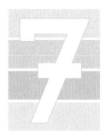

Weight Gain with Chronic Illness and Impaired Liver Detoxification

ɪɪɪ Chronic Illness and Impaired Liver Screening Questionnaire

Circle the number of any statement that applies to you.

1. I started gaining weight after I contracted a chronic illness.

2. I have a chronic illness (e.g., chronic fatigue syndrome, fibromyalgia, rheumatoid arthritis).

3. I frequently feel exhausted.

4. I frequently feel sick all over, like having the flu or mono.

5. I am very sensitive to medications.

6. I am very sensitive to smoke, chemicals, or fumes in the environment.

7. I am taking or have in the past taken a lot of prednisone, non-steroidal anti-inflammatory drugs (NSAIDS, such as Motrin, Advil, ibuprofen), antibiotics, antidepressants, or other medications.

8. My illness causes me to be quite sedentary.

9. I have had frequent yeast infections (including thrush).

Answer Key: If you have circled four items, it is possible that impaired liver detoxification is contributing to your weight problem; if you have circled five or more items, it is likely that significant issues with impaired liver detoxification are contributing to your weight problem and switched metabolism.

ııl Glossary of Medical Terms Used in Chapter 7

detox beverage: A hypoallergenic, rice-based protein formula containing selected nutrients that augment liver detoxification.

GALT: An acronym for gut-associated lymphoid tissue; 60 percent of the body's immune response comes from GALT.

leaky gut syndrome: A gut condition characterized by increased intestinal permeability, which occurs when the wall of the small intestine is damaged. This permeability allows toxins made by bacteria, yeast, and/or parasites to leak out of the gut into systemic circulation, where they can cause symptoms of inflammation, compromise the immune system, and impair liver detoxification. In addition, large molecules of partially digested foods can escape from a permeable gut.

liver detoxification: The process by which the liver protects us from toxins in the environment and in our diet that circulate in our bloodstream. These toxins come from our food, water, and air; on a more subtle level, these toxins can come from toxins manufactured in our bodies, microbes, and prescription drugs.

ııl A Common Story

I wish I had a dollar for every time in my medical career I have heard the following: "Dr. Rigden, my weight was always normal until I contracted my chronic medical condition. Since then, I have gained weight steadily and can't seem to stop gaining."

Geri's Story

When Geri came to our office at age 49, she explained that she had weighed 135 pounds for many years until she became ill, suffering chronic fatigue, depression, anxiety, and chronic stress over the previous eight months. During that time she gained 23 pounds. In addition she had developed high blood pressure, with readings as high as 161/90 (nl: 130/80). She was taking three medications for her symptoms and was feeling terrible, with low energy. Her weight had not responded to several popular commercial diet programs.

Initial Tests and Measurements
Height: 5 feet, 3 inches
Weight: 159.4 pounds
Waist circumference: 35 inches
Blood pressure: 161/90
Body fat: 27 percent

Extensive lab work was within normal limits.

Assessment
Geri suffered from the following conditions:

1. chronic fatigue with chronic high stress, anxiety, and depression
2. hypertension
3. overweight

Recommendations
We recommended that Geri apply the following program:

1. Initiate modified elimination diet, with the use of a hypoallergenic detox beverage designed to promote improved liver detoxification twice daily.
2. Begin walking 30 minutes daily.

3-Month Follow-Up
Geri's weight is 133 pounds, her blood pressure is 137/82 (off all meds), her waist circumference is 32 inches, and her body fat is 24.5 percent.

1-Year Follow-Up
Geri is now off all medications and has no symptoms of chronic fatigue. She is working out 60–90 minutes five times a week. She states, "The liver detoxification program helped me to lose 24 pounds, normalized my blood pressure, and got me off my medications. I haven't felt this good in years."

Summary

	INITIAL	FINAL
Weight	159.4 pounds	135.2 pounds
Waist circumference	35 inches	31 inches
Blood pressure	161/90	137/82
Body fat	27 percent	21 percent

ıl Inactivity and Prescription Medications

Two factors that often influence a remarkable weight gain are inactivity and prescription medications. Most chronic illnesses, such as chronic fatigue syndrome (CFS), fibromyalgia (FM), and lupus, greatly limit activity levels. Common sense recognizes that a sedentary lifestyle sustained for months or years is a significant factor in weight gain. A person burning off 200 fewer calories each day due to chronic illness will, in a year, burn off 73,000 fewer calories, for a weight gain of almost 20 pounds!

Unfortunately, a number of popular pharmaceutical drugs promote weight gain. Many people who have taken these drugs for a long period of time have not had a clue that these drugs have made weight management difficult, if not impossible. The following is a list of some of the most problematic drugs.

Table 7.1: Medications That May Cause Weight Gain

Anticonvulsants	Valproic acid, carbamazepine
Antidepressants	Tricyclic antidepressants, including Elavil (amitriptyline); monoamine oxidase (MAO) inhibitors (Nardil); selective serotonin reuptake inhibitors (SSRIs) including Paxil and Zoloft, Remeron
Anticancer agents	Arimidex for breast cancer is an example
Corticosteroids	Prednisone, for example
Insulin	Up to a 17-pound weight gain can occur in an intensive three-month treatment course
Lithium	Gains can be up to 22 pounds or more in 6 to 10 years
Oral contraceptive agents	Ethinylestradiol leads to dose-dependent increase in body fat

(cont'd.)

Table 7.1: Medications That May Cause Weight Gain (cont'd.)

Oral hypogly-cemic agents (sulfonylureas)	Usual weight gain is more than 11 pounds during 3 to 12 months of treatment
Antipsychotics	Haloperidol, loxapine, olanzapine, and clozapine are the most likely to cause gain

ıl Impaired Liver Detoxification

When it comes to the difficult weight-control problems of chronically ill overweight patients with switched metabolism, the most significant cause frequently is impaired liver detoxification.

> Patients with chronic illness gain weight due to decreased activity and prescription drug side effects. Impaired liver detoxification is frequently the most significant factor in this problem.

As often happens in science, I learned this surprising fact while doing clinical research on the relationship between chronic fatigue syndrome/fibromyalgia and liver detoxification; at the time I had no thought about any possible relationship to weight gain. Further research about liver detoxification helped to clarify this relationship.

ıl Why Do We Accumulate Toxins?

Our modern lifestyle has drastically changed the chemistry of the environment in which we live. There is ample documentation of increased toxicity in our food, air, and water. In addition, chronic illnesses often are connected to the production of toxic chemicals that cause inflammation and oxidative stress. Moreover, many medications are metabolized in the liver, and, in effect, they can function as toxins. Unfortunately, many of us promote an increase of our own toxin levels with excessive alcohol intake, smoking, and drug use.

> We live in an environment of potentially toxic exposures to food, air, and water. In addition, chronic illnesses often produce toxins internally that cause symptoms in the body. Pharmaceuticals can also be potentially toxic compounds. The liver must handle all of these toxins.

ıl Phase 1 and Phase 2 Liver Detoxification

In its simplest form, liver detoxification involves two steps (see Figure 7.1). In phase 1, a toxin initially enters the p-450 cytochrome system, and is broken into smaller fragments. These fragments then progress to phase 2, where they are connected to molecules like glutathione, glycine, and sulfate. This process creates a new, nontoxic molecule that can be excreted from the body in the bile, urine, or stool.

One or both detoxification phases can be inefficient, overworked, or overloaded. A particularly damaging combination in an ill person is an excessive overload of toxins coming in phase 1, with an inefficient phase 2 conjugation process. Some scientists believe this combination may be the cause of marked environmental sensitivities and idiosyncratic drug intolerances and interactions that characterize many CFS/FM patients.

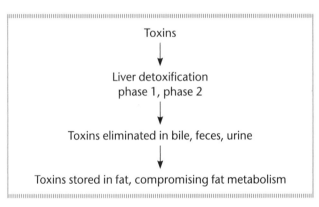

FIGURE 7.1. The body's detoxification system

ıl Liver Detoxification Test

Researchers at the Functional Medicine Research Center in Gig Harbor, Washington, in conjunction with our efforts in Arizona, have tested more than 200 CFS/FM patients in research protocols for the adequacy of their liver detoxification. This test involved administering a calculated amount of caffeine, acetaminophen (Tylenol), and aspirin and collecting urine over a designated time period. Our research indicates that 80 percent of CFS/FM patients have significantly impaired liver detoxification. Furthermore, as patients improve clinically, serial testing of their liver detoxification capacity shows corresponding improvement. Another important clinical result of this research was the conclusion that patients who are very ill with severe toxic symptoms must undergo liver detoxification very slowly and gradually. It is always preferable first to reduce total body toxins and inflammation before initiating liver detoxification. For example, if leaky gut syndrome, a condition that increases systemic toxins released from the gut, was found, a gut program to reduce toxins was necessary prior to the liver detoxification. We will discuss leaky gut syndrome later in this chapter.

ı Surprise!

We expected that applying a protocol for liver detoxification consisting of a cleansing diet and the use of a rice-based, hypoallergenic medical food containing specific nutritional supplements to augment liver detoxification would lead to improved liver detoxification and correspondingly healthier functioning by the patients. Indeed, our clinical research confirmed these results.[1] What surprised us was that many patients who had gained significant weight and had been mired in switched metabolism for months or years after contracting CFS/FM suddenly began to lose weight rapidly. Many of them continued to lose weight well after the three-week liver detoxification program. This observation left us very happy but temporarily confused. Eventually, we developed the following hypotheses, which we believe explain this interesting phenomenon.

ıl How Liver Detoxification Helps Weight Loss

Compromised liver detoxification and the subsequent buildup of liver and system toxins leads to compromised fat metabolism. It is almost as if our bodies perceive toxin buildup as a threat and implement defense strategies, including the hormonal and molecular message to our fat metabolism, "Hold on. We're under siege!" A liver detoxification program employing a hypoallergenic, rice-based protein formula containing nutrients that support and augment liver detoxification, combined with an elimination diet, can effectively lower toxin levels. This, in turn, leads to improved fat metabolism and weight loss.

Compromised liver detoxification and the subsequent buildup of liver and system toxins impair fat metabolism. A liver detoxification program with a hypoallergenic, rice-based protein formula containing nutrients that support and augment liver detoxification, combined with an elimination diet, effectively lowers toxin levels; this leads to improved fat metabolism and weight loss.

ıll The Role of Leaky Gut Syndrome

Leaky gut syndrome, or increased intestinal permeability, occurs when the wall of the small intestine is damaged. This permeability allows toxins made by bacteria, yeast, and/or parasites to leak out of the gut into systemic circulation, where they can cause symptoms of inflammation, compromise the immune system, and impair liver detoxification. In addition, large molecules of partially digested foods can escape from a permeable gut. The symptoms produced by excessive intestinal permeability may be limited to the gastrointestinal tract or may involve the entire body. They can include irritable bowel syndrome, fatigue and malaise, headache, joint and muscle pain, and skin eruptions. Common causes of damage to the cells lining the gut, leading to this increased permeability, may include harmful bacteria, unhealthy balance of good versus bad bacteria, yeast, parasites, and chronic inflammation from food allergens, medications, and alcohol.

Leaky gut syndrome, or increased intestinal permeability, occurs when the wall of the small intestine is damaged.

ıll Leaky Gut Syndrome and Liver Detoxification

People with chronic illnesses frequently have both leaky gut syndrome and impaired liver detoxification. When this is the case, the leaky gut syndrome, a constant source of systemic toxicity, needs to be resolved before liver detoxification can be improved.

ıl Causes of Leaky Gut

- stress
- infections
- some diseases
- medications
- food allergies
- hormones
- parasites
- alcohol
- drugs

- yeast overgrowth   - bacterial imbalance   - tobacco
- endotoxins produced by microbes

Leaky gut syndrome is often confused with irritable bowel syndrome and is not recognized as a factor that can influence weight. It can be a major source of chronic toxicity that is often overlooked. See Figure 7.2 to help visualize and understand the concept of leaky gut syndrome.

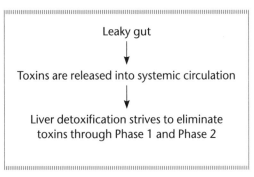

FIGURE 7.2. Leaky gut syndrome

To better elucidate leaky gut syndrome, let's talk about GALT, tennis courts, and bricks.

ıı GALT

Sixty percent of the body's immune response comes from gut-associated lymphoid tissue, or GALT. Therefore, when dealing with health problems in which the immune system is compromised, such as chronic fatigue syndrome, it is logical to work on restoring and improving gut functioning.

ıı Tennis Courts

Imagine that somehow you could remove the intestines from the body and spread their absorptive surface on the ground. Astonishingly, this tissue would cover the area of a tennis court! Populating this tennis court are two to three pounds of bacterial flora, and we would hope the ratio of this population would favor the healthy microbes. You can imagine the effort it would require to cleanse even a quarter of a tennis court of inappropriate microbial inhabitants!

ıl Bricks

Observe how the junctions between the bricks in a well-constructed new house are tightly compacted with mortar. Even a severe rainstorm cannot cause a leak. Now compare this structure to an old, much-neglected brick house. The bricks are crumbling and the mortar is decaying. Notice how a rainstorm readily causes leakage. Similarly, the intestinal lining in a person with leaky gut syndrome contains cells that are not tightly connected, allowing leakage of toxins out of the gut into the body.

Fifty percent of patients with CFS/FM have leaky gut syndrome. For liver detoxification in these patients to be effective, it is necessary first to treat leaky gut syndrome and reduce the toxic load on the liver. Identifying and treating leaky gut syndrome are preliminary steps to help CFS/FM patients break through switched metabolism and begin losing weight.

ıl The Four "Rs" Program

A damaged intestinal lining with increased permeability (leakage) can be confirmed by the lactulose/mannitol test. In this test, the patient drinks a sweetened solution containing the largest-known sugar molecule, lactulose, and the smallest sugar molecule, mannitol. After assessing the urine for the amounts of these molecules that were able to pass through the gut, one can establish this diagnosis. Indirectly, one can infer leaky gut syndrome if a stool sample confirms the presence of excessive amounts of pathogenic bacteria, a poor balance of healthy and unhealthy bacteria (bacterial dysbiosis), yeast overgrowth, and/or parasites.

In general, the 4R approach, which stands for remove, replace, reinoculate, and repair, is very effective in dealing with leaky gut syndrome. The patient must first remove toxins and dietary provocateurs. Pathogenic bacteria, yeast, and parasites are thus eradicated or reduced. Foods that may trigger an inflammatory response are eliminated. Replace, the second R, often

> Leaky gut syndrome is present in 50 percent of patients with chronic illness and switched metabolism. For liver detoxification to be successful in improving fat metabolism in these patients, it is first necessary to repair the leaky gut syndrome.

includes the addition of digestive enzymes, fiber, and hydrochloric acid to restore homeostasis to the GI tract. Reinoculate implies the restoration of a healthy balance of flora in the gut. Lactobacillus and bifidus bacteria are often needed; fructooligosaccharides to help cultivate a nurturing environment for the healthy balance of flora in the gut. Repairing the damaged mucosal lining requires a number of nutrients, including L-glutamine, pantothenic acid, zinc, and essential fatty acids.

ιl Achieving Effective Liver Detoxification

The basics of the liver detoxification program are simple. For four weeks, consume an elimination diet (similar to the modified elimination diet in Chapter 6) while also utilizing, on a daily basis, a hypoallergenic, rice-based protein powdered beverage with additional selected nutrients that augment liver detoxification.

These nutrients include glutathione, N-acetyl cysteine, glycine, alpha-lipoic acid, and B vitamins.

> The basics of the liver detoxification program are:
>
> 1. Consume an elimination diet for four weeks.
>
> 2. Utilize on a daily basis a hypoallergenic, rice-based protein formula containing selected nutrients that augment liver detoxification.

Although this program seems simple, you need to know several things in order to undertake it successfully. Planning, preparation, and knowing what to expect are essential for good results. For example, most individuals experience transient reactions to the program during the first several days of detoxification. In other words, you may feel worse initially. Symptoms may include mild headaches, fatigue, muscle aches, or changes in bowel habits. Please don't be discouraged! Usually the symptoms are minor and temporary. The first benefit often is unusually sharp and clear cognitive function, followed by steady improvement of physical symptoms and, in many cases, weight loss. It is important to note that if you normally consume a significant amount of caffeinated beverages or sugars, you may experience withdrawal headaches if you discontinue them all at once. I suggest that you gradually decrease your intake of caffeine and sugar over five to seven days, before you start the 28-day program.

It is common early in the detoxification process to experience mild, transient symptoms like headaches, fatigue, muscle aches, and bowel changes. These symptoms can be minimized by gradually decreasing caffeine and sugar intake prior to the program.

ıl Getting Started

The program is divided into three steps:

Step 1: Initial Clearing (days 1–6): During Step 1 you will eliminate potentially allergenic foods (see Table 7.2) while you slowly increase the intake of the nutritional support product to augment liver detoxification.

Step 2: Detoxification (days 7–21): During Step 2 you will continue to follow a hypoallergenic diet, along with three servings a day of your nutritional support product.

Step 3: Reintroduction (days 21–28): During Step 3 you will slowly reintroduce the foods you eliminated in Step 2 into the dietary plan and slowly decrease the intake of your nutritional support product. Careful attention should be paid to symptoms or weight gain as you reintroduce foods. These reactions could be important clues regarding food allergies or intolerances. Keep careful records.

Table 7.1. Recommended Schedule for Reintroducing Foods in Step 3

Days 21 and 22	Gluten-containing grains, one serving daily
Day 23	Dairy products, one serving
Day 24	Eggs, one serving
Day 25	Orange, one serving
Day 26	Corn, one serving
Day 27	Peanuts, one serving
Day 28	Soy, one serving

After day 28, discuss and coordinate with your medical provider regarding further additions.

ıı General Program Guidelines

Try to adhere strictly to the diet and recommendations regarding your detox support beverage. The following food plan is identical to the plan presented in Chapter 6 for food allergies.

Table 7.2. Liver Detox Food Plan

FOOD GROUP	ALLOWED	AVOID
Meat, Fish, Poultry	Chicken, turkey, lamb Cold-water fish such as salmon, halibut, mackerel, trout	Red meat, cold cuts, frankfurters, sausage, canned meat
Legumes	All legumes, dried peas, and lentils	Soy products
Eggs	Egg replacer (made from potato starch or flax seeds)	Eggs, cholesterol-free egg substitutes
Dairy Products	Milk substitutes such as rice milk, nut milks	Milk, cheese, cottage cheese, yogurt, ice cream, cream, nondairy creamers, soy milk
Starch	White or sweet potato, arrowroot, rice, tapioca, buckwheat, millet, gluten-free products	All gluten-containing products, including pasta, all corn, and corn-containing products
Bread/Cereal	Any made from rice, quinoa, amaranth, buckwheat, teff, millet, potato flour, tapioca, arrowroot, or gluten-free flour-based products	All made from wheat, oat, corn, pelt, kamut, rye, barley, gluten-containing grains, corn-containing products
Vegetables	All vegetables, preferably fresh, frozen, or freshly juiced	Creamed vegetables or those made with prohibited ingredients
Fruits	Unsweetened fresh, frozen, freshly juiced, or water-packed, canned fruits, excluding oranges	Fruit drinks, ades, cocktails, citrus, strawberries, and dried fruits preserved with sulfites
Soup	Clear, vegetable-based broth, homemade vegetarian soup, made with ground chicken or turkey, bean soup	Canned or creamed soup Any soups containing glutenous flours or chili grains

(cont'd.)

Table 7.2. Liver Detox Food Plan (cont'd.)

FOOD GROUP	ALLOWED	AVOID
Beverages	Freshly prepared or un-sweetened fruit or vegetable juice, pure water, noncitrus herbal tea, diluted fruit juices	Milk, dairy-based products, coffee, tea, cocoa, Postum, alcoholic beverages, soda pop, sweetened beverages, citrus drinks
Fats/Oils	Cold, expeller pressed, unrefined, light-shielded canola, flax, olive, grape-seed, pumpkin, sesame, and walnut oil, salad dressings made from allowed ingredients	Margarine, shortening butter, refined oils, salad dressing and spreads
Nuts/Seeds	Almonds, cashews, flax seeds, pecans, pumpkin seeds, sesame, squash seeds, sunflower seeds, walnuts, nut/seed butters, pistachios	Peanuts and peanut butter
Sweeteners	Brown rice syrup, fruit sweeteners, agave nectar, Stevia	Brown and white sugar, honey, evaporated cane juice, maple syrup, corn syrup, molasses

1. Try to consume all of the recommended servings of your powdered beverage. (The detox beverage used in our office is UltraClear-Plus, made by Metagenics Inc. We also use Ultra-Clear-Plus pH in these programs.) This product contains important ingredients for the nutritional support of your body's detoxification processes. I recommend the following progression in beginning to consume the detoxification product and ramping it up to full strength, followed by tapering down. Days 1 and 2: one-half scoop twice daily; days 3 and 4: one scoop twice daily; days 5 and 6: two scoops twice daily; days 7 to 21: two scoops three times daily; days 22 to 24: two scoops twice daily; days 25 to 26: one scoop twice daily; days 27 to 28: one scoop daily.

How to Take Your Detox Beverage

Days on Detox Program	Scoops per Day
1 and 2	½ scoop daily
3 and 4	1 scoop twice daily
5 and 6	2 scoops twice daily
7–21	2 scoops three times daily
22–24	2 scoops twice daily
25–26	1 scoop twice daily
27–28	1 scoop daily

2. Select fresh foods whenever you can. Fruits and vegetables grown without pesticides and herbicides are desirable, if available.

3. The preferable sources of animal protein on the program would be cold-water fish (e.g., salmon, halibut) or free-range raised chicken, turkey, or lamb. Trim visible fat and prepare by broiling, baking, stewing, grilling, or stir-frying. Avoid shellfish, which is more likely to cause an allergic reaction.

4. In regard to other nutritional products, supplements, and medications, follow the advice of your health-care practitioner. In some cases, it may be dangerous to discontinue or decrease certain prescriptions.

5. Use purified, distilled, or mineral water, or diluted juice to mix with the powdered beverage. Avoid mixing with fruit drinks or cocktail drinks that contain added sugar.

6. Drink at least 2 quarts (64 ounces) of plain, purified, distilled, or mineral water each day.

7. Strenuous or prolonged exercise should be reduced during the program to allow your body to cleanse more effectively.

8. When possible, choose a four-week period for the program in which you do not plan to travel, have company, or participate in stressful events.

9. Before starting the program, take time to plan your menus and shopping lists. Good planning is often the key to a successful program!

Examples of Daily Menus
Example: Day 4

Breakfast	1 scoop of detox powdered beverage Crispy brown rice cereal with rice or almond milk, sliced fruit, cinnamon
Snack	Sliced fruit sprinkled with sunflower seeds or chopped pecans
Lunch	Large mixed green salad with chopped walnuts, Balsamic Mustard Vinaigrette (see recipe on page 215) Bean soup 1 scoop of detox powdered beverage
Snack	Raw veggies with ¼ cup hummus
Dinner	Vegetarian chili or Turkey Chili (see recipe on page 220) Mixed green salad with olives, sliced onion, garbanzo beans, Balsamic Mustard Vinaigrette (see recipe on page 215)
Snack	Fruit cup of strawberries, banana slices, chunks of pineapple, pieces of apple, and raw cashews

Example: Day 8

Breakfast	2 scoops of detox powdered beverage Apple
Snack	Rice cakes and almond butter
Lunch	2 scoops of detox powdered beverage Vegetable rice soup One small-to-medium chicken breast Peach or pear
Snack	2 scoops of detox powdered beverage
Dinner	4–6 ounces of salmon Baked sweet potato *or* brown rice Dinner salad of mixed greens, avocado, basic salad dressing Stir-fried asparagus *or* steamed broccoli
Snack	2 scoops of detox powdered beverage

■||||||||||||||||||||||||||||||■

In conclusion, impaired liver detoxification and leaky gut syndrome have become more prevalent over the past twenty years because of our changing environment. Given the challenges we face in our food, water, and air supplies, in addition of the common practice of polypharmacy, it is amazing more people do not suffer from these conditions.

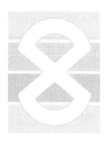

Dealing Effectively with Emotional Eating

Okay, admit it. You have read the first seven chapters of this book, but you are still spinning your wheels. You are frustrated and can't quite pinpoint what is holding you back from the success you so deeply desire. If this is the case, my experience indicates you may be plagued by issues involving emotional eating. Emotional eating almost always leads to inappropriate eating. Without realizing it, you may be caught in a vicious cycle of "living to eat," not "eating to live." There is no simple answer for this tendency. However, since it seems that everyone from Dr. Phil to Oprah Winfrey has an opinion on this subject, I would like to share some techniques and thoughts that have helped many of my patients for more than 20 years. Consider this chapter as a smorgasbord or cafeteria of ideas. Pick and choose what seems to fit you and give it your best shot. After all, you have nothing to lose, except those unwanted pounds!

> Emotional eating almost always leads to inappropriate eating. Without realizing it, you may be caught in a vicious cycle of "living to eat," not "eating to live."

ɪɪɪ Research on the Ineffective Lifestyle Syndrome

After conducting extensive research on why people in weight-loss programs dropped out, I published my findings in the *Bariatrician*, the medical journal of the American Society of Bariatric Physicians for weight-loss specialists.[1]

I catalogued numerous reasons patients became bogged down in a complex weight-loss project. I named the most frequent behavioral and psychosocial variables the "Ineffective Lifestyle Syndrome." The problem areas included excessive passivity (being "too nice"), poor self-image, feeling controlled by external rather than internal events, invalid or rigid belief systems, compulsive overeating, stress eating, depression, and being victims of abuse. Obviously, some readers will have several of these difficulties.

Ineffective Lifestyle Syndrome and What to Do about It

PROBLEM	REFER TO THIS SECTION IN THIS CHAPTER	PAGE
Compulsive overeating	"Help for Compulsive Eaters"	page 198
Depression	"Depression"	page 203
Excessive passivity (being too nice)	"Are You Too Nice?"	page 189
	"The Vicious Cycle of Being Passive and Manipulated"	page 190
	"Techniques to Improve Assertiveness"	page 191
External versus internal control	"Three Important Lists"	page 192
Invalid or rigid belief systems	"The Importance of a Positive Mental Attitude"	page 183
	"Getting in Touch with Denial"	page 189
	"Weight-Loss Mind Games"	page 199
Poor self-image	"Do You Like Yourself?"	page 184
	"Techniques to Improve Your Self-Image"	page 186
	"Your Positive Attributes List"	page 187
Stress overeating	"Daily Relaxation"	page 178
	"Assess Stress in Your Life"	page 180
Victims of abuse	"Victims of Abuse"	page 206

This chapter will address these problems and offer practical tips and solutions. There is no one technique or strategy that cures all and that is needed by every reader. As a result, consider the chapter a potpourri of ideas from which you can pick and choose.

ılı Daily Relaxation

In this busy, hustle-bustle world it has become increasingly important to include a daily relaxation period. Relaxation implies learning to silence all physical muscular tension, as well as to attain calm and tranquility. True relaxation can be measured with physiological parameters in laboratories. It correlates with specific changes that scientists have documented. Relaxation skills can be taught, and they improve with practice. The physical changes measured during relaxation correlate with increased health and improved mental and physical functioning in the body.

Hundreds of articles published in scientific journals show that 20 minutes a day spent in true relaxation can lead to the following positive physical changes: decreased blood pressure, decreased heart rate, decreased respiratory rate, and decreased perspiration. It can also increase alpha brain waves (associated with a feeling of inner calm or peace), increase endorphins (chemicals in the brain and nervous system that help ease depression and increase pain tolerance), decrease anxiety, and increase energy. Twenty minutes a day of true relaxation has been shown to be more restorative and refreshing than deep sleep.

You could employ any number of different techniques to promote successful daily relaxation. One is having a daily "mini vacation." Mini vacations involve a type of pleasant, guided visual imagery that can help you get into a meditative state.

ıl Mini Vacations (How to Relax)

Pick a time and place that will be quiet and uninterrupted for at least 20 minutes. This technique is most effective when you use it daily. Start by sitting in a comfortable chair or lying down on your back. Begin by consciously letting go of the various muscle groups of your body. Do not expend too much effort in doing this. Try to pay attention to each part of your body and release the tension there. You will find you can always voluntarily relax to a certain degree. Starting at the top of your head, stop frowning and let your forehead relax. Ease up on the tension in your jaw. Then let your hands, your arms, your shoulders, and your legs become a little more relaxed. Spend about five minutes doing this and then stop paying attention to your muscles. This is as far as you are going to try to go by conscious control. Now move into the mini-vacation relaxation exercises.

Mini Vacation #1

In your mind's eye, see yourself in a prone position with two very heavy concrete legs. See these heavy concrete legs sinking far down into the mattress from their sheer weight. Now imagine your arms and hands are made of concrete. They, too, are very heavy and are sinking down into the bed and exerting tremendous pressure against the bed. In your mind's eye, see a friend come into the room and attempt to lift your heavy concrete legs. He takes hold of your feet and attempts to lift them, but they are too heavy for him. He cannot do it. Repeat this imagery with your arms, neck, and head.

Mini Vacation #2

Imagine your body is a life-size marionette. Your hands are tied loosely to your wrists by string. Strings loosely connect your forearms to your upper arms and your upper arms to your shoulders. Your feet, calves, and thighs are also connected by strings. Your neck is one very limp string. The strings that control your jaw and hold your lips together have slackened and stretched to such an extent that your chin has dropped down loosely against your chest. All the strings that connect your various body parts are loose and limp, and your body is sprawled loosely across the bed.

Mini Vacation #3

Imagine your body as a series of inflated balloons. Two valves open in your feet, and the air begins to escape from your legs. Your legs begin to collapse and continue until they are just deflated rubber tubes lying flat against the bed. Next a valve is opened in your chest, and as the air begins to escape, your entire trunk begins to collapse limply against the bed. Continue the same imagery with your arms, head, and neck.

Mini Vacation #4

Go back in memory to some relaxing and pleasant scene from your past. There is always some time in everyone's life when he or she felt relaxed, at ease, and at peace with the world. Pick your own relaxing picture from your past and call up detailed memory images. You may remember relaxing in the sun on a beach. How did the sand feel against your body? Could you feel the warm sun touching your body, almost as a physical presence? Was there a breeze? Were there gulls on the beach? The more details you can remember and picture to yourself, the more successful you will be.

Daily practice of these mini vacations will cause these mental pictures or memories to become increasingly clear. The effect of practice is cumulative. Practice will strengthen the tie-in between mental image and physical sensation, and you will become more and more proficient in relaxation.

ııl Assess Stress in Your Life

We all have stress. In fact, without some stress our lives would be boring and we could not function at our best. However, when stress in your life reaches the saturation point, it can turn into a monster, feeding on itself to the point that it makes you a temporary or permanent victim. It can also trigger you to eat inappropriately in a futile attempt to comfort yourself and relieve the stress. Many people are in such a rut that they are in denial about this stress level. Perhaps the stress level has been so high for so long that they have become accustomed to it and do not realize how it affects them. You can assess the level of stress in your life by looking at the Holmes and Rahe Life Stress Rating Scale below.[2] This psychological tool has been validated among numerous ethnic and social groups. Take time to fill out this Life Stress Questionnaire. The instructions are self-explanatory.

Life Stress Questionnaire

During the past two years, have you had any of the following things happen to you? If so, simply circle one of the numbers following those items (and only those items) that apply to you. Circle only one number after each event that has occurred in your life recently.

LIFE STRESS QUESTIONNAIRE

LIFE EVENT	SLIGHT	MODERATE	GREAT
1. Change in social activities	10	15	20
2 .Change in sleeping habits	10	15	20
3. Change in residence	10	20	30
4. Change in work hours	15	20	25
5. Change in church activities	15	20	25
6. Tension at work	20	25	30
7. Small children in the home	20	25	30
8. Change in living conditions	20	25	30
9. Outstanding personal achievement	25	30	35
10. Problem teenager(s) in the home	25	30	35
11. Trouble with in-laws	25	30	35
12. Difficulties with peer group	25	30	35
13. Son or daughter leaving home	25	30	35
14. Change in responsibilities at work	25	30	35
15. Taking over a major financial responsibility	25	30	35
16. Foreclosure of mortgage or loan	25	30	35
17. Change in relationship with spouse	30	35	40
18. Change to different line of work	30	35	40
19. Loss of a close friend	30	35	40
20. Gain of a new family member	35	40	45
21. Sex difficulties	35	40	45
22. Pregnancy	35	40	45
23. Change in health of family member	40	45	50
24. Retirement	40	45	50
25. Loss of job	45	50	55
26. Change in quality of religious faith	45	50	55
27. Marriage	45	50	55
28. Personal injury or illness	45	50	55

(cont'd.)

LIFE STRESS QUESTIONNAIRE (cont'd.)			
	POINT VALUE		
LIFE EVENT	**SLIGHT**	**MODERATE**	**GREAT**
29. Loss of self-confidence	55	60	65
30. Death of a close family member	50	60	70
31. Injury to reputation	50	60	70
32. Trouble with the law	55	65	75
33. Marital separation	55	65	75
34. Divorce	65	76	85
35. Death of spouse	80	100	120
36. Other: (invalid in family; drug or alcohol problem, etc.) _____	_____	_____	_____
Total of three columns	_____	_____	_____

Scoring System:
Greater than 300: highly significant life stress
200–300: significant life stress
150–200: moderate life stress
Less than 150: low life stress

The general idea is that as life stress change units increase, the risk of health problems rises accordingly and, in my experience, the likelihood of stress eating also increases. If your score is less than 150 life stress change units, the likelihood that you are at increased risk for a health breakdown is very low. If your score is between 150 and 200 units, there is a mildly increased risk of health challenge. If your score is between 250 and 300 units, there is a moderately high risk of a significant health problem. If your score is greater than 300, you are at major risk of a significant health crisis; moreover, it creates a high-stress environment that increases the likelihood of stress eating. If you have a high score, you should consider ways to cope constructively with the stress in your life. Make this stress a stepping-stone for increased coping ability and strength, and do not allow it to control your life. If your high stress level is correlated with an exacerbation of obesity or weight problems, it may be necessary to seek stress-management counseling from a behavioral health specialist. Many of the ideas in the rest of this chapter may also be helpful.

ııl The Importance of a Positive Mental Attitude

We have talked a lot about your physical diet. It is also important to have an increased awareness of your mental diet. Many people are prone to mental indigestion. It is easy to have our minds and attitudes blocked by a constant influx of negative thoughts and feelings. One does not have to look far to see that the radio, television, and newspapers can overwhelm us day after day with reports of tragedies and bad news. Our friends and coworkers, overwhelmed by their own problems, may be unable to give us positive energy. This constant bombardment of negativity can make living a joyful, hopeful life seem almost impossible. Therefore, every day we need to have some kind of uplifting or inspirational experience to fill our lives and this void. A positive mental attitude is essential in dealing with stress, but developing this attitude requires commitment and strategies. I encourage you to start your own inspiration file, including books, articles, CDs, cassette tapes, and other materials, which you can access on a daily basis. You can use these resources as an antidote or substitute for inappropriate stress eating.

If reading doesn't excite you or you don't have time to read, you might consider the wealth of outstanding CDs and tapes that are now available. Your local library has a wide variety of books on tape or CD. You can listen to these messages daily while you get ready for work, perform routine household tasks, or drive your car.

A tendency to start taking life too seriously may also indicate trouble with high stress levels. If it has been quite a while since you have been able to smile or laugh, particularly to laugh at yourself, you may be falling into a negative rut. Humor and laughter are healing. The well-known author Norman Cousins healed himself of an "incurable" illness by the vigorous application of laughter

> A positive mental attitude is very important. Begin to develop your own inspiration and humor files, including books, articles, CDs, tapes, and cartoons, which you can access readily. You can use these resources as an antidote or substitute for inappropriate stress eating.

therapy. Although totally bedridden with what his doctors had described as an incurable illness, he started to experience pain relief and have improved blood tests as soon as he began laughing at old comedy movies and reruns of *Candid Camera*. Scientific studies have shown that people suffering from ulcers and excessive stomach acid production literally cannot make excessive acid if they are smiling or laughing. Along with your inspiration file, begin to keep your personal humor file. Accumulate funny stores, anecdotes, cartoons, articles, tapes, and other materials that you can access readily to give your life and its problems a lighter touch.

ıl Do You Like Yourself?

Assess Your Self-Image

How would you rate your self-image? Circle the number of any of the following statements that applies to you.

1. I am uncomfortable with my appearance.
2. I often feel inferior or "put down."
3. My reason for wanting to lose weight is not primarily for myself and my inner needs.
4. Eating and weight problems interfere with optimal expression of my femininity (masculinity).
5. I feel insecure in my personal relationships.
6. I lack self-confidence.

Answer Key: If you circled the numbers of four or more of these statements, it is likely that you have a poor self-image that may be holding you back. Three positive answers certainly indicate a possibility that you need to improve your poor self-image.

It is very difficult to be successful at weight reduction when you have a negative self-image.

Self-image is defined as the composite of thoughts and feelings a person has integrated throughout a lifetime. A poor self-image leads to unsuccessful, self-defeating behaviors and often to negative, self-fulfilling prophecies. This self-defeating behavior, in turn, leads to habitually negative self-talk and feedback, reinforcing a negative self-image. Poor self-image as a "loser" in the weight-loss game may cause a person to feel unloved or unaccepted. Ask yourself the question: "Do I love myself?" For many overweight individuals, the answer is a resounding "No!" As part of a negative concept, many obese individuals dislike their bodies. Plagued by poor self-esteem, these individuals are obsessed with comparing themselves to others and with the opinions of others. For example, when I was 65 pounds overweight, I remember deliberately turning the lights off or turning away from the mirror when I was shaving because I so disliked my appearance. In fact, I even hated to walk past clean windows because I might see my reflection in the glass.

> Self-image is defined as the composite of thoughts and feelings that a person has integrated throughout a lifetime. A poor self-image leads to unsuccessful, self-defeating behavior and often to negative self-fulfilling prophecies.

A typical trait of self-dislike is the tendency to tear oneself down. Examples include giving credit to others when it rightfully belongs to you, rejecting compliments, making up excuses for looking nice, and so forth. A lack of self-love, and treating oneself as unimportant, makes it easy to remain the same. Subconsciously, as long as one feels unworthy of the money, time, and effort required to lose weight, there is just no point in trying to grow or become better, healthier, and happier.

> A typical trait of self-dislike is the tendency to tear oneself down.

Some psychologists feel a lack of self-acceptance begins at a young age and leads to compulsive eating. Perhaps a person feels her mother did not show as much love as she wished she had. Another might feel he could never live up to his father's expectations. Someone might feel his or her inadequacies prevented winning the approval of family and friends. Such an individual's life might be plagued by feelings of never running fast enough or performing adequately. As he or she continues to strive to do more and be better, the person enters into a maladaptive behavior cycle in which he or she turns to food for comfort. For the moment, the poor self-image may be soothed by food, but shortly afterward the brief good feeling is replaced by guilt and remorse, and the same old struggle resumes.

ıl Techniques to Improve Your Self-Image

Have you ever noticed that you have a continuous dialogue going on within yourself? We call that dialog self-talk or feedback. We are consistently making and storing little tapes in the memory banks of our minds, much like a computer does. These tapes can be either positive or negative. An example of a positive tape would be, "That's excellent, John. You are doing a super job. You're going to make it this time and nothing will stop you." An example of a negative tape would be, "Oh boy, John, you've blown it again. You are a real failure." For many areas of our lives in which we have performed below our expectations, we have made literally thousands of these negative tapes. How we habitually talk to ourselves affects our self-image.

Make Positive Mental Attitude Cards

To improve your self-image, I recommend that you start immediately to work on the area of self-talk. Begin with 3 × 5-inch cards, which we call PMA, or Positive Mental Attitude cards. These cards should include short, positive statements in the first person. The statements should be exciting, personal, and phrased to indicate that dynamic things are about to happen. The following PMA cards might be helpful as examples.

> I react to all events in my life today with positive optimism. Challenging situations with food are great opportunities for growth!

> I eat to live, not live to eat, so every day I feel more confident about my eating habits!

> I am a calm, confident, peaceful,
> poised person. I have a ready smile,
> laugh, and sense of humor.

Post these messages in your kitchen, bedroom, bathroom, office, or car. Repeat them to yourself, with enthusiasm, several times a day. Start replacing your negative tapes with positive ones.

Mirror Technique
A related technique that yields great results is to post the following sign on your bathroom mirror:

> _____ (your name),
>
> a positive attribute I have that I appreciate is
>
> _____.

Start your day with this positive self-affirmation each morning before you enter into your daily activities. Each day you must repeat a different trait.

ıl Your Positive Attributes List

Another helpful technique to boost your self-image is to keep a bed-side notebook in which you enter your positive attribute list. Each night, before retiring, add several items to your list. Look at yourself the way a caring friend or sibling would. This is not narcissism. It is merely a way of getting in touch and reminding yourself of the many positive attributes you may not often think about. Many of our patients find it meaningful to repeat a short prayer of thanks after adding to their list before they go to sleep.

My Positive Attributes List

Example: I am a sincere and caring friend.

Example: I am dependable.

Example: I am a good mother (or father) and am devoted to my family.

Example: My arms and legs are strong and in good shape.

Example: I have a good sense of humor.

Example: I am working on self-improvement.

1. _____

_____

2. _____

_____

3. _____

_____

4. _____

_____

5. _____

_____

6. _____

_____

7. _____

_____

8. _____

_____

9. _____

_____

10. _____

_____

ꞁꞁ Getting in Touch with Denial

I often see patients who are out of touch with the reality of their daily choices and behaviors and how these things can impact their health and weight. This type of denial can occur even in the most intelligent and highly educated individuals. It may be a defense because the person is not ready to embark on serious personal inventory or change. This denial may occur because we are in a rut and/or may be living such a hectic life that we do not take the time for introspection. Whatever the cause of denial, it needs to be eradicated for the person to commit to long-term change. The following are some simple but very helpful exercises to move past denial.

Techniques to Recognize and Move Beyond Denial

1. Write yourself a letter explaining in detail why you believe you have a weight problem. Discuss issues regarding accepting personal responsibility for the weight problem.

2. Make up a list of "What I dislike about me and my life" and "Who and what is to blame." Discuss this list with someone you trust.

3. Work daily with the following three questions:

    1. Why do I want to eat?

    2. Has eating really ever solved a problem in my life?

    3. What are alternate activities to eating when I am under stress?

4. If a particular problem is holding you back from progressing with your weight-control program, consider the SOLVE approach: State your problem. Outline what it is and is not. List approximately ten alternatives and select the best three. Visualize the long-term consequences of achieving those three. Evaluate your solution and implement it.

ꞁꞁ Are You Too Nice?

Is it possible to be too nice or "too sweet"?

Learn to Be Assertive

Answer the following questions honestly:

1. It is very important to me to please other people.
2. I often put other people's needs ahead of my own.
3. I have difficulty in saying no and really meaning it.
4. I am a "doormat."
5. I have difficulty expressing my feelings.
6. I give in to other people.
7. Other people easily manipulate me.

If you answered yes to four or more of these questions, it is probable that you are too passive. If you answered yes to three or more of these questions, you may be too passive. What does this mean? And what does it mean to be more appropriately assertive?

As a nonassertive individual, you may often be so concerned with pleasing other people and being "nice" that you often find yourself feeling guilty or being manipulated. It can be very difficult for a passive overweight or obese person to say no and really mean it when it comes to food choices.

ılI The Vicious Cycle of Being Passive and Manipulated

Does this sound like you?

- Friends or relatives manipulate you to conform to their interests and desires.
- You feel guilty if you do not give in to their urgings.
- You deviate from your best intentions and eat inappropriately.
- You feel more guilt.
- You become anxious and depressed.

These feelings reinforce your low self-esteem and make you think, "I knew I was no good" or "I'll always be a failure." You give yourself negative feedback and adopt an attitude of self-deprecation.

All of this leads back to your deviating from your best intentions and eating inappropriately.

ııl Techniques to Improve Assertiveness

Many known techniques can help you cope with manipulators. I learned three of my favorites from the late bariatric pioneer, Dr. Peter Lindner.

The Parrot Technique

The Parrot Technique involves persistent unruffled repetition of the same words, without deviation from what one wants to say, until the manipulator exhausts his bag of tricks.

Feeling Talk

Feeling Talk enables you to say how you really think and feel. Express honest feelings without fear of reprisal. Take charge of the conversation! Listen for cues to information other people give about themselves, and prompt them to reveal more of their true feelings.

Agreeing with Criticism

Agreeing with Criticism allows you to agree with the truth, principle, or possibility of criticism—not what is implied. Carefully listen to the individual's exact words and respond only to what is actually being said. Don't justify, deny, or find fault, and thus furnish a "striking surface" to the manipulator.

Assertive wisdom maintains that as a human, you are entitled to the same rights as anyone else. It is proper and desirable for you to decide what is best for you and your body and health and to take full responsibility for your actions. Remember, only you can take this responsibility. No one else, even those who love you, can do this. As you increase your assertiveness, it is well to remember that to err is human, and it is your privilege to say, "I don't know." It is okay to change your mind when you feel like it. Nobody is perfect!

ıll Three Important Lists

Many of us manage the days of our demanding, busy lives by making "to-do" lists. The first list is usually "All the things I have to do today," which may be long, as well as urgent. Examples could be work, a doctor's appointment, meetings, personal hygiene and grooming, meal preparation and eating, and so on. The second list contains "All the things I sort of have to do today." This list could include activities such as car and house maintenance, laundry, paying bills, correspondence, and the like.

You also need to be aware of three important lists that can help you overcome emotional eating. These are the alternate activity list, the nurturing activities list, and the rejuvenating activity list.

My Alternate Activity List
Alternate activities are those activities that fulfill the three criteria of (a) keeping you busy; (b) competing with eating; and (c) being readily available. This list should be posted on your refrigerator where you can easily see it and work with it when you feel like eating inappropriately. It can be a big asset if you have trouble with inappropriate eating in the evening. Obviously, activities like reading, watching TV, working on the computer, or hiking in the mountains do not fulfill all three of these criteria. Also, be aware that these activities do not have to be grandiose or expensive. Some examples that patients have shared with me include taking a shower, reorganizing a closet, vacuuming the rugs, and washing the car. We will help you get started with the list on the next page. Strive to include at least ten items.

My Alternate Activity List
Example: Practice a musical instrument.
Example: Weed the garden.
Example: Clean my desk.

1. _____

_____

2. _____

_____

3. _____

_____

4. _____

_____

5. _____

_____

6. _____

_____

7. _____

_____

8. _____

_____

9. _____

_____

10. _____

_____

My Nurturing Activity List

Many of us eat for comfort. After a long, hard day of work and dealing with family issues, we may feel the need for nurturing later in the evening. But we may be very tired and fall into the rut of reaching for what is always there and readily available—food! Granted, when you eat you may feel some comfort that lasts a few minutes, but the feeling is fleeting, and it is not long before you have to eat something more. As you embark on a program that limits eating except to satisfy true biological hunger, you may feel as though you have given up a dear friend, in the form of food, which you counted on for pseudo-nurturing. Therefore, one of the key lists in re-inventing yourself and your relationship with food is to develop other nurturing activities that replace food. Examples shared by patients include a warm bath, a back rub, and listening to soothing music. Start your own nurturing list and post it where it can be readily seen. Remember, these activities cannot involve food. On the following page is a list to get you started. Making your own list is more difficult than you might imagine, because our culture typically associates food with the idea of nurturing.

My Nurturing Activity List
Example: foot rub
Example: manicure
Example: massage

1. _____

_____

2. _____

_____

3. _____

_____

4. _____

_____

5. _____

_____

6. _____

_____

7. _____

_____

8. _____

_____

9. _____

_____

10. _____

_____

My Rejuvenating Activities List
By the time you get to the third list, unfortunately, you may be running out of time and energy. This list contains activities that speak to your soul, things you love to do, and things that rejuvenate you and make you whole. The items on this list are very important in enabling you to function as a balanced, effective, healthy person. From a health perspective, it is key to having a strong immune system and becoming revitalized. This list should include quality time alone as well as dates or quality time with your significant other (your spouse without the children, for example). Think of this as your "sanity list." Examples my patients gave me include calling a loved one on the phone, spending time drawing or painting, and bird watching. Start your own sanity list today and begin to rearrange your schedule to include some blocks of time necessary for your personal rejuvenation.

My Rejuvenating Activities List
Example: walking in nature
Example: photography
Example: brushing my dog

1. _____

_____

2. _____

_____

3. _____

_____

4. _____

_____

5. _____

_____

6. _____

_____

7. _____

_____

8. _____

_____

9. _____

_____

10. _____

_____

ıl Help for Compulsive Eaters

Most compulsive eaters have tried every diet they have ever heard of or read about. They may have lost weight on each one of them, only to regain the lost weight and more besides. They often are obsessed with thoughts of food and their next snack or meal. Binges are frequently followed by feelings of guilt and remorse. Feast and famine and weight yo-yos frequently are the modus operandi of the compulsive eater. Compulsive eaters often describe being out of control with their eating. They are not aware of what they are doing and what they are eating. Compulsive eating may take up a large amount of time, planning binges, worrying about one's body, thinking about eating, and strategizing about how different life will be when one is thin.

> Compulsive eaters often are obsessed with thoughts about food and the next snack or meal. They describe being out of control with their eating and have an "all-or-nothing" approach to eating behavior.

The compulsive eater can benefit from employing satiety strategies and oral gratification techniques.

ıl Satiety Strategies

Whether the problem stems from years of mental programming or from biochemical uniqueness, most compulsive eaters cannot handle feeling empty. When the stomach registers empty, something seems to snap, and irreversible eating binges occur. The compulsive eater simply cannot stop with one cracker or cookie. Realistically, the entire package of goodies is at high risk. It is important that the compulsive eater accept this difference and feel comfortable with the idea that they cannot do well by eating once or twice a day, or by trying to eat as little or as infrequently as possible. This is a sure way to trigger the feast/famine cycle that has prevented consistent results in the past. It is preferable to have a series of satiety strategies that you can comfortably employ at danger times, such as late morning, midafternoon, after work, or late in the evening.

My Strategic Snacks for Satiety

The list on the next page includes a number of snacks to have available. Always precede your snack by drinking 16 ounces of water and follow the snack with a piece of sugar-free chewing gum. Feel free to add your own ideas to the list.

Strategic Snacks for Satiety

- raw vegetable plate
- soup
- fruit plate
- hard-boiled egg
- 12 raw almonds
- 2 tablespoons pumpkin or sunflower seeds
- nonsugary protein drink or protein bar
- herbal tea, a diet soft drink, or coffee, accompanied by 3 ounces of low-fat turkey or a piece of fruit
- apple slices, with 2 teaspoons of natural nut butter
- large green salad with Balsamic Mustard Vinaigrette (see Recipe on page 215)

Oral Gratification Techniques

Many times the perception that we need to eat is not triggered by true biological hunger. Instead, this urge or craving can be satisfied by alternatives such as sucking on a cinnamon stick, chewing on a toothpick, or chewing sugarless gum. Delaying the compulsive need to eat by 20 to 30 minutes often causes the urge to pass. Always try to have these aids on hand to help promote your sense of being in control.

ıl Weight-Loss Mind Games

Individuals who are not succeeding in controlling their weight may employ a number of different mind games. These games, while understandable, get in the way of effective weight management and must be identified and understood.

ıl It's Not Fair

We are all individuals with unique biochemistries. Because some of us have been given different genetics, a slower metabolism, or a different way of distributing fat, we are quite correct in saying, "It's not fair!" But whoever said life was fair? We all have our own assets and liabilities according to our unique genetic potential. With discipline and hard work, our liabilities can, in part, be neutralized and overcome. It is silly to waste time and energy complaining that it's not fair that you have a weight problem. The point is that you do, and something must be done about it.

ıı I'm a Failure

Typically, people feel that once they have faltered on their weight-management program or have a history of alternating between losing and gaining weight on diet programs that they are "failures," and they label themselves as such. Actually, nothing could be further from the truth. Observe sports teams. Just because it has a bad first quarter, a football team doesn't condemn itself as a failure. Players can eliminate mistakes, fumbles, penalties, and bad strategies and go on to dominate and win the game. Similarly, we can learn from our mistakes and failures and react with the idea that "to falter is not to fail." The only way a person can truly be a failure at the weight-loss game is to quit trying at all.

ıı Unrealistic Expectations and Goals

Many weight-loss patients may be doing very well in the eyes of their physician, but because they had unrealistic expectations, perhaps due to the media or to advertisements, they feel disappointed and disillusioned. Others may start a weight-management program with goals that are totally unrealistic. For example, one of our patients who was 5 feet 10 inches tall and who had reduced her weight from 180 pounds to 145 pounds was sad because she could not approach the 5 foot, 10 inch, 118-pound stature of model Christie Brinkley.

ıı Spouse Competition

Competition with a spouse in weight loss can really undermine the female half of a marital team. Because of basic physiological differences, there is no way the female body can lose weight as rapidly and efficiently as the male. For example, one couple in my practice undertook the exact same diet and exercise program. In eight weeks, the husband lost 27 pounds and the wife lost 18 pounds. Over the long haul, both can be equally successful, but at differing rates of weight loss. Sometimes, on the other hand, the success of one spouse threatens the resolve of the other. If the slower-reducing spouse has a poor self-image, he or she may fear losing the love of his or her spouse who is improving in health and appearance. As a result, the less successful spouse may actually begin to sabotage the successful spouse's program.

ıı It Doesn't Count If...

Many people play an interesting little mind game that causes them to follow a food program or diet religiously except...if they are flying, driving, eating out, on a weekend holiday, on vacation, at their bridge club, and so on. Somehow, their mind-set is that calories consumed on these occasions do not count the same as calories consumed in the regular daily routine. Unfortunately, it only takes one or two major indiscretions in a week to undo five or six days of self-discipline and commitment.

ıı There Is a Magical Shortcut

Deep down inside we all want to find a quick-fix weight-loss program. Unethical weight-loss advertisements and programs in the media further enhance this fantasy. In fact, most crash diets only present the illusion of quick weight loss. This counterfeit weight loss is actually made up of muscle and fluid, not the fat tissue the individual seeks to lose. Unfortunately, weight lost by this counterfeit means quickly comes back after the crash diet is finished.

ıı The Faster I Lose Weight the Better

The rate of weight loss is greatly overrated. As a person evaluates a weight-loss program, more important considerations are the program's safety, long-term success rates of participants, and whether the weight lost is fat or fluid and muscle. There are no data to support the idea that the faster the weight loss, the greater the level of long-term success for the patient. In fact, the data would seem to indicate the opposite. Remember, in weight loss, the tortoise often beats the hare.

ıı Self-Pity/Martyrdom

Many individuals who undertake a weight-loss program really get into the "poor me" scenario. A way to win this weight-loss mind game is to talk not about paying the price of success, but about enjoying the process of success. Reflect on how much you enjoy feeling and looking better, and feeling and looking younger. Focus on how much you enjoy the surprised look on the faces of folks who have not seen you in some time. Observe how much you enjoy your new agility, energy, and ability to participate fully in the activities of your life.

ıI I Don't Need to Exercise

One of the greatest mistakes of overweight individuals is to insist on trying to overcome a weight problem without exercise. Almost every study on this subject indicates that exercise not only facilitates weight loss but also greatly improves long-term success in weight maintenance after weight reduction. The numerous benefits of exercise on one's health include improved coronary risk factors and antistress and antidepressant benefits. In addition, the combination of exercise with diet is much more likely to ensure a good body appearance after the weight loss. Dieting without exercise often just accentuates a pear shape, particularly in women.

ıI Dieting: All or Nothing

An all-or-nothing attitude toward dieting easily undermines a basically successful weight-loss program. The typical story might run something like this. A man has been on a good weight-loss program for two weeks; however, while dining with co-workers at a Mexican restaurant, he has some nachos. He then rationalizes that "Since I have blown my diet, I might as well live it up." Subsequently, he consumes a 3,000-calorie Mexican dinner and continues to gorge himself the rest of the week. Obviously, attempting to follow a program even at an 80 percent level is far preferable to zero percent compliance. A better strategy is to forsake all-or-nothing thinking and realize that "Although I may not be perfect, I will strive to learn from my mistakes and correct them as soon as possible."

ıI If I Eat Only Once a Day

Some patients come to us after experiencing what they describe as the "last straw." That is, they could not lose weight even though they had cut back to only one meal daily. Unfortunately, they did not understand that if one is prone to slow metabolism, this strategy often backfires. In this scenario of deprivation, it is as if the body's metabolism decides to prevent its owner from starving and triggers physiologic effects leading to very efficient calorie storage, at the expense of burning calories. Spreading 1,000 calories over three to four meals a day yields results that are superior to an equal 1,000 calories consumed on the one-meal-a-day approach.

ıl I Don't Need Help

Your ego may not like to admit that you need help to achieve weight loss. This weight-loss mind game contrasts with the behavior patterns of successful individuals in many aspects of their lives. Most professionals at the top of their fields are glad to receive expert help and coaching with their problems. Professional golfers, for example, frequently take their personal coach on tour with them. If anything at all seems a little out of line, they work on it vigorously with their coach. While the desire for independence in achieving weight-loss results is understandable, it is more important to be open and receptive to expert advice. Even highly sophisticated dietitians and physicians with weight-management problems can benefit by working closely with another professional.

ıl Depression

I have found that evaluating obesity problems in patients with depression and/or those who are on antidepressant medications can raise unique problems. In my clinical experience, patients who actively manifest symptoms of depression and are not stabilized on a program for their depression cannot do well with attempts at weight loss. On the other hand, it is certainly reasonable for these patients to consider a weight-loss program after their depression has become stabilized.

Depression can be insidious and is often missed in a clinical diagnosis. Even though you may not feel sad or unhappy, if you are unable to enjoy things that used to give you pleasure and seem to be "stuck in neutral," consider talking to a professional for an evaluation. The Beck Depression Inventory, developed by Dr. Aaron Beck at the University of Pennsylvania Medical School, has become a gold standard for family physicians to use for the screening of clinical depression in their patients.

Beck Depression Inventory

On this questionnaire are groups of statements. Please read the entire group of statements of each category. Then pick out the one statement in that group which best describes the way you feel today, right now! Circle the number beside the statement you have chosen. If several statements in the group seem to apply equally well, circle each one. Be sure to read all the statements in each group before making your choice.

A.	3	I am so sad or unhappy that I can't stand it.
	2	I am blue or sad all the time and I can't snap out of it.
	1	I feel sad or blue.
	0	I don't feel sad.
B.	3	I feel that the future is hopeless and that things cannot improve.
	2	I feel I have nothing to look forward to.
	1	I feel discouraged about the future.
	0	I am not particularly pessimistic or discouraged about the future.
C.	3	I feel I am a complete failure as a person (parent, husband, wife).
	2	As I look back on my life, all I can see is a lot of failures.
	1	I feel I have failed more than the average person.
	0	I feel I have the average number of failures.
D.	3	I am dissatisfied with everything.
	2	I don't get satisfaction out of anything anymore.
	1	I don't enjoy things the way I used to.
	0	I am not particularly dissatisfied.
E.	3	I feel as though I am very bad or worthless.
	2	I feel quite guilty.
	1	I feel bad or unworthy a good part of the time.
	0	I don't feel particularly guilty.
F.	3	I hate myself.
	2	I am disgusted with myself.
	1	I am disappointed in myself.
	0	I don't feel disappointed in myself.
G.	3	I would kill myself if I had the chance.
	2	I have definite plans about committing suicide.
	1	I feel I would be better off dead.
	0	I don't have any thoughts of harming myself.
H.	3	I have lost all of my interest in other people and don't care about them at all.
	2	I have lost most of my interest in other people and have little feeling for them.
	1	I am less interested in other people than I used to be.
	0	I have not lost interest in other people.

(cont'd.)

Beck Depression Inventory (cont'd.)

I.	3	I can't make any decisions at all anymore.
	2	I have great difficulty in making decisions.
	1	I try to put off making decisions.
	0	I make decisions about as well as ever.
J.	3	I feel that I am ugly or repulsive looking.
	2	I feel that there are permanent changes in my appearance and they make me look unattractive.
	1	I am worried that I am looking old or unattractive.
	0	I don't feel that I look any worse that I used to.
K.	3	I can't do any work at all.
	2	I have to push myself very hard to do anything.
	1	It takes extra effort to get started at doing something.
	0	I can work about as well as before.
L.	3	I get too tired to do anything.
	2	I get tired from doing anything.
	1	I get tired more easily than I used to.
	0	I don't get any more tired than usual.
M.	3	I have no appetite at all anymore.
	2	My appetite is much worse now.
	1	My appetite is not as good as it used to be.
	0	My appetite is no worse than usual.

Scoring System:

Greater than 12: Very significant depression

8–12: Significant depression

(Source: Developed by Dr. Aaron Beck, University of Pennsylvania Medical School)

Because of difficulties with fluctuating lithium levels, fluid shifts, and electrolyte imbalances, I do not treat outpatients who are on lithium with diets that use protein drinks. These patients can be more safely treated with a food-only dietary approach. Tricyclic antidepressants like amitriptyline (Elavil) are notorious for causing carbohydrate food craving and weight gain. Selective serotonin reuptake inhibitors like (SSRIs), fluoxetine (Prozac), sertraline (Zoloft), and paroxetine (Paxil) seem to cause weight gain after six months of use. There are some exceptions in which I have seen patients start to gain weight almost immediately while on these drugs. The two best antidepressant choices in obese, depressed patients in my experience have been Effexor and Wellbutrin. Research and my own experience indicate they are weight-neutral.

> If you are clinically depressed, it is important to stabilize this condition before you seriously tackle your weight problem. If an antidepressant medication is indicated, ask your physician to discuss with you the best options to avoid the common side effect of weight gain.

ı11 Victims of Abuse

I cannot stress strongly enough that if you presently live in a relationship involving abuse, alcoholism, or adultery, it is imperative for you to seek psychological help with the goal of establishing a more psychologically healthy environment before you can tackle your weight problem. Similarly, if you have never psychologically dealt with a history of early episodes of physical, emotional, or sexual abuse as a youth or teen, it is also imperative for you to seek help. The effects of these painful and often catastrophic events are beyond the scope of this book and my expertise. I can tell you, however, that I have frequently referred unsuccessful weight-management patients who were also victims of abuse to therapists who specialized in these areas; after they received help from a qualified therapist over a period of time, many of these same patients have expressed much gratitude and in some cases have gone on to lose significant weight and live much healthier lives.

Conclusion

"He who labors diligently need never despair;
for all things are accomplished by diligence and labor."

— MENANDER (342–292 BC)

"One can never consent to creep
when one feels an impulse to soar."

— HELEN KELLER (1880–1968)

ıll It's about Time!

You have just read many pages of new information designed to help you reinvent yourself. No matter what your age, no matter how many times you have met futility in the past, it is never too late to initiate a successful campaign. The key is to realize that if you have a metabolic condition that makes traditional calorie counting likely to fail, you need to adopt a new paradigm. You have read numerous case studies that are inspiring; you, too, can try a new approach and enjoy the positive rewards and results. But there will never be a totally ideal time to embark on your new program, so do not procrastinate! If not now, when?

ıll Time to Review

Before you plunge in, quickly review Chapters 1 and 2. Do you know your cholesterol, blood sugar, triglycerides, blood pressure, and waist circumference results? What are your reasons for wanting to manage your weight successfully? List them and sign your personal contract as a symbol of your commitment. State realistic plans for exercise and water intake and plan how you will keep daily records.

ıl What Are My Metabolism Issues?

Review Chapters 3 to 8 and your responses to the screening questionnaires. Your questionnaire scores should give you a good idea of your
metabolic issues; specifically, you have screened yourself for tendencies to carbohydrate sensitivity, metabolic syndrome, hormonal imbalances, food hypersensitivities, and chronic illness/impaired liver
detoxification. Also review your responses to the life stress questionnaire in Chapter 5 and the depression inventory in Chapter 8.

ıl Get Professional Help

Now it is important for you to obtain professional help for the monitoring, education, and motivation that you need to sustain permanent success. I belong to two groups of caring, knowledgeable medical
professionals that I encourage you to consider. The physicians in the
American Society of Bariatric Physicians (www.asbp.org) and the Institute of Functional Medicine (www.fxmed.org) should be on your
radar screen.

ıl What Do You Have to Lose?

In conclusion, I want to thank you for reading this book. Why not
try a new metabolic-oriented weight-management approach for
sixty days? If it works—and it has already worked for hundreds of
so-called "hopeless cases"—you will feel younger and better, improve your appearance and self-esteem, be able to stop some or all of
your medications, and add years of healthy living to your life. What
is the worst-case scenario? If it doesn't work for you, you will only be
60 days older and medically unchanged. That is no disaster! Really,
what have you got to lose but some unwanted pounds!

Recipes

The recipes in this section are suitable for consumption by people of all metabolic types.

SOUPS

Cucumber Soup

1–2 medium seedless cucumbers
1 shallot or garlic clove
1½ tablespoons fresh dill
1 cup buttermilk
1 cup plain low-fat yogurt
Salt and pepper, to taste

Purée cucumbers, shallot or garlic clove, and dill in a food processor or blender. Add buttermilk and blend again. Pour into a serving bowl and whisk in yogurt. Season to taste with salt and pepper and add more dill if needed. Cover and chill for 1–2 hours.

Makes 4 servings.

Oven-Baked Lentil and Split Pea Soup

½ cup lentils
½ cup split peas
5 cups vegetable or chicken broth
1 cup each sliced carrot, celery, red bell pepper, and onion
1 bay leaf

1 teaspoon ground cumin

Salt and pepper, to taste

¼ cup low-fat plain yogurt, optional

Rinse lentils and peas. In an oven-proof baking dish or Dutch oven, combine all ingredients except yogurt. Cover and bake at 350 degrees for about 2 hours, until all ingredients are tender. If you wish soup to cook faster, bring to a boil on top of stove, cover and simmer for about 1 hour. Remove bay leaf and garnish each serving with a spoon of yogurt, if desired.

Makes 4–6 servings.

Roasted Winter Squash and Apple Soup

Large butternut squash, about 2–3 pounds, peeled, seeded, and cut into 1–2 inch pieces

1 large onion, peeled and cut into 6–8 large chunks

3 garlic cloves, peeled

2 tart apples, peeled, quartered, and cored

2 tablespoons olive oil

Dash mild chili powder

4 cups vegetable or chicken broth

Preheat oven to 400 degrees. In a large roasting pan, combine the squash, apple, onion, garlic, and oil. Season with salt and sprinkle with chili powder. The more chili powder, the more "bite." Roast for 45 minutes, stirring every 10–15 minutes, until veggies are tender and lightly browned. In a food processor, combine half of the roasted veggies with 2 cups broth and puree until smooth. Repeat with the remaining veggies and heat over medium heat in a saucepan, stirring occasionally. Add more broth as needed if soup is too thick. Add more salt and chili powder if desired for personal taste.

Makes 4–6 servings.

White Beans and Greens Soup

2 cloves garlic, minced

1 large onion, chopped fine

1 tablespoon olive oil

1 carrot, scrubbed and diced

2 cans (15 ounce cans) white beans, rinsed and drained

4 cups of vegetable or chicken broth or water

½ teaspoon thyme

¼ teaspoon sage

1 bay leaf

1 bunch of fresh greens, such as escarole, kale, collards, chard, or bok choy, thinly sliced, with tough veins removed

Salt and pepper to taste

Grated parmesan, as an optional garnish

Over medium heat, sauté onion in olive oil for 2 minutes. Add carrot and garlic, and continue to sauté for 2 more minutes. Add beans and broth or water, spices, and greens. Simmer for 20–30 minutes. Remove bay leaf and discard. Garnish with grated parmesan, if desired.

Makes 6 servings.

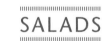

SALADS

Cucumber Yogurt Salad

1 English cucumber, thinly sliced

½ cup red onion, thinly sliced

1 clove garlic, minced

3 tablespoons chopped fresh dill

¼ teaspoon coarse salt

1 cup plain yogurt

2–3 teaspoons white wine vinegar

Combine cucumber, onion, garlic, dill, salt, and yogurt.

Stir in white wine vinegar and adjust seasoning for salt. Add freshly ground pepper, to taste. Garnish with a dusting of fresh dill and serve immediately.

Makes 4 servings.

Grains and Beans Salad

½ cup wheat berries
½ cup quinoa (rinsed twice in a strainer)
¼ cup millet
1 package (10 ounces) frozen lima beans, defrosted
1 cup chopped bell pepper (red, yellow, or green)
1 cup diced celery
⅓ cup currants
¼ cup freshly chopped parsley
½ teaspoon dried thyme
½ teaspoon dried dill weed (or 1 tablespoon fresh dill)
Salt and pepper to taste
Roasted Garlic Vinaigrette (see recipe on page 215)

Boil water in a medium saucepan. Add only the wheat berries. Reduce heat, cover, and simmer for 40 minutes. Then add rinsed quinoa and millet, cover, and simmer for 15 minutes more, until all grains are tender. Drain.

In a large serving bowl, combine the grains with the Roasted Garlic Vinaigrette and mix well. Cover and chill for 3–4 hours or overnight.

Cook lima beans according to package instructions. Drain and add to the chilled grains, along with the remaining ingredients.

Makes 6–8 servings.

Tropical Salad

1 can (16 ounces) hearts of palm, cut into ½ inch slices
1 can (12 ounces) artichoke hearts, packed in water, halved
3 stalks celery, thinly sliced
2 whole avocados, diced

Dressing:

¼ cup red wine or balsamic vinegar

1½ teaspoon Dijon mustard

1 small shallot, minced

1 clove garlic, minced

1 teaspoon each dried tarragon and parsley

Salt and pepper to taste

¾ cup olive oil

Put all ingredients, except olive oil, into a jar. Shake well. Add olive oil and continue to shake until well mixed. Gently mix dressing into the vegetables. Serve on a bed of lettuce.

Makes 6–8 servings.

Chicken Salad with Green Beans and Walnuts

Dressing:

3 tablespoons vinegar (white wine or balsamic)

1 tablespoon Dijon mustard

Dash each of salt and freshly ground pepper

¼ cup extra virgin olive oil

In a small jar, shake together first 4 ingredients. Add oil and shake until well blended.

Salad:

1½ pounds fresh green beans, steamed until crisp tender, and cooled

2 boneless (skinless) chicken breasts, baked or poached, and cooled (or use leftover chicken or turkey)

1½ cups coarsely chopped walnuts or pecans

⅓ cup chopped fresh basil or parsley

¼ teaspoon freshly ground black pepper

Combine salad ingredients in a large serving bowl. Drizzle with dressing and toss until all ingredients are well coated. Serve immediately.

Makes 4–6 servings.

Barley Lentil Salad

1 cup dried lentils, rinsed
2 cups chicken or vegetable broth
1 cup uncooked pearl barley
2¾ cups water
½ red onion, chopped
⅓ cup chopped fresh parsley, plus extra for garnish
½ cup lemon juice
¼ cup olive oil
Salt and freshly ground pepper, to taste
2 garlic cloves, minced

Combine lentils and broth in a large saucepan over medium-high heat and bring to boil. Reduce heat and simmer about 10 minutes or until liquid is absorbed, stirring occasionally. Stir in barley and water and bring to a simmer. Cook 15–20 minutes, until liquid is absorbed, stirring occasionally. Transfer mixture to a large bowl and add remaining ingredients, stirring well to combine. Cool to room temperature, then cover and chill about 1 hour prior to serving. Garnish with fresh parsley, if desired.

Makes 6 servings.

Snow Pea and Asparagus Salad

Dressing:

Grated zest of 1 lemon
¼ cup lemon juice
2 teaspoons Dijon mustard
Ssalt and freshly ground pepper, to taste
½ cup extra virgin olive oil

Salad:

2 teaspoons olive oil
1½ pounds fresh asparagus, sliced into 1-inch pieces
1½ pounds sugar snap peas, remove ends and strings
2 tablespoons minced fresh dill

1–2 hard-cooked eggs

Salt and pepper, to taste

In a small jar, shake together all dressing ingredients, except olive oil. When well mixed, add olive oil and shake again. Set aside while fixing the vegetables.

Stir-fry asparagus and peas in olive oil until tender but not soft, about 3–5 minutes. Allow to cool. Combine vegetables with dill, salt and pepper, and toss with the dressing. Serve garnished with chopped hard-boiled eggs.

Makes 6–8 servings.

SALAD DRESSINGS

Roasted Garlic Vinaigrette

2–3 garlic cloves

3–4 tablespoons balsamic vinegar

2 tablespoons chopped shallots or green onion

1 tablespoon Dijon mustard

4–5 tablespoons olive oil

Peel garlic and place in a shallow baking pan or on a cookie sheet. Bake uncovered at 350 for 15–20 minutes until golden and soft in the center. In a blender, combine roasted garlic with remaining ingredients, except olive oil. Cover and blend for 10 seconds. While the blender is running, slowly drizzle in olive oil and mix until well blended.

Makes enough to toss one salad.

Balsamic Mustard Vinaigrette

½ cup extra-virgin, cold-pressed olive oil (or ¼ cup each flax and olive oils)

3 tablespoons balsamic vinegar

(any vinegar is fine, but this has the richest flavor)
2–3 tablespoons water
1 teaspoon Dijon mustard
1–3 cloves fresh garlic (use either whole pieces for flavor
or crushed for a stronger taste)
Salt and pepper to taste
Oregano, basil, parsley, tarragon, or any herbs you like, fresh or dried
(oregano and basil are typical of Italian dressings)

Place vinegar, water, and mustard into a jar with a secure lid and shake well to incorporate mustard.

Add oil and remaining ingredients and shake well again.

Store in refrigerator and shake well before using. (Dressing will congeal when refrigerated and will need 5–10 minutes at room temperature to reliquify.)

(Amounts are approximate—you may wish to use more or less of certain ingredients to your personal taste). Keep a jar in the refrigerator at work and one at home.

MAIN COURSE

Coconut Curried Shrimp

1½ pounds peeled and deveined shrimp
1 tablespoon minced fresh ginger or 1 teaspoon ground ginger
2 garlic cloves, minced
1 tablespoon sesame oil
1 red or green bell pepper, diced
1½ cups fresh broccoli florets, broken into small pieces
½ to 1½ teaspoons Thai red or green curry paste
(the more you use, the spicier!)
1 teaspoon curry powder
1 can (15 ounces) coconut milk
2 tablespoons soy sauce

¼ cup chopped fresh basil or 1 tablespoon dried basil

2 cups cooked brown rice

Heat sesame oil in a large skillet or wok over medium-high heat. Add shrimp and ginger. Cook 3–4 minutes, stirring. Remove shrimp and set aside (they are not yet fully cooked). Add bell pepper, broccoli, curry paste, garlic, and curry powder to skillet or wok and cook for 3–4 minutes, stirring constantly. Lower heat to medium and add coconut milk and soy sauce. Cook for 4–5 minutes more, stirring often. Add shrimp back and cook another 2 minutes until shrimp are no longer pink. Do not overcook or shrimp will be tough. Remove from heat and stir in basil. Serve immediately with brown rice.

Makes 4 servings.

Baked Italian Omelet

8 eggs, beaten

1 cup part-skim ricotta

½ cup 1 percent or non-fat milk

½ teaspoon dried basil

¼ teaspoon salt

¼ teaspoon pepper

1 package (10 ounces) frozen spinach, thawed and squeezed dry

1 cup chopped plum tomatoes

1 cup shredded part-skim mozzarella

½ cup scallion, thinly sliced

1 cup chopped turkey or ham

Preheat oven to 325 degrees. Combine eggs and ricotta in a large bowl. Stir in milk and seasonings. Fold in spinach, tomato, mozzarella, scallion, and turkey or ham. Spread evenly in a greased baking dish (2–3 quarts).

Bake for 30–35 minutes or until a knife inserted near the center comes out clean. Allow to stand for 10–15 minutes.

Makes 6–8 main dish servings.

Mushroom/Tofu Stew

2 tablespoons olive oil
1 medium onion, diced
1 red bell pepper, diced
1 teaspoon dried tarragon
2 cloves garlic, minced
1 pound mushrooms, cleaned and sliced
1 can (15 ounces) garbanzo beans (chick peas)
1 pound package extra-firm tofu, cut into cubes
½ cup chopped fresh basil
2 cups cooked brown rice or barley

Sauce:
2 tablespoons Dijon mustard
1 tablespoon tamari (lower sodium soy sauce)
2 tablespoons Worcestershire sauce
¾ cup dry red wine

Mix the ingredients for the sauce and set aside. Heat 1 tablespoon olive oil in a large pan or wok. Sauté onion over medium heat until softened. Add bell pepper, tarragon, and garlic and continue to cook for about 10 minutes. Remove from pan. Add remaining tablespoon of oil to the same pan and add sliced mushrooms. Sauté over medium-high heat until juices begin to release, about 5 minutes. Add the onion/pepper mixture back to the pan and stir until well mixed.

Add the sauce to the onion/pepper/mushroom mixture in the pan. Stir to mix well and add ½ cup water. Simmer for about 15 minutes, stirring occasionally. Add tofu and garbanzo beans and simmer for another 15–20 minutes. Garnish with fresh basil.

Serve with cooked brown rice or barley.

Makes 4 servings.

Wild Rice with Shrimp and Fennel

½ cup uncooked wild rice, well rinsed

¼ teaspoon salt

1 pound shrimp, shelled and deveined(fresh or frozen)

¾ cup sliced fennel

1 cup white kidney beans (cannelini)

1 small red or yellow bell pepper

2 green onions

¼ cup slivered almonds for garnish (optional)

Dressing:

3 tablespoons olive oil

1 tablespoon white wine vinegar

1 tablespoon lemon juice

2 teaspoons Dijon mustard

1 clove garlic, minced

Salt and pepper to taste

Bring 1½ cups water to a boil in a heavy saucepan. Stir in rice and salt, and return to boil. Reduce heat and simmer, covered, 50–60 minutes or until kernels begin to puff open (cook only 40–45 minutes for a chewier texture). Uncover and fluff with fork. Simmer, uncovered, five more minutes. Drain excess liquid as needed.

Mix dressing ingredients with a wire whisk (or shake in a jar). In a serving bowl, combine shrimp, rice, fennel, beans, bell pepper, and green onions, and toss with dressing. Garnish with slivered almonds, if desired.

Makes 4 servings.

Note: You may use 1 pound of frozen, peeled, and deveined shrimp. Some packages are already cooked and you need only defrost in the refrigerator. Others need to be cooked following package directions. Be careful not to overcook, as shrimp will become tough.

Cooking shrimp: Bring two quarts of lightly salted water to a boil. Turn off the heat and add the shrimp to the water. Allow to sit in water about 3 to 5 minutes, or until done. It is important for shrimp to be cooked gently and not for too long. Check by cutting one shrimp in half. If its flesh is opaque throughout, it's done. Drain immediately and proceed with recipe.

Salmon or Tuna Wrap

2 cans (7 ounce cans) wild salmon or chunk-lite tuna or
1 pound fresh tuna or wild salmon
1 teaspoon olive oil (if using fresh fish)
1 teaspoon Herbs de Provence or ¼ teaspoon each thyme,
rosemary, basil, and sage
8 ounce container hummus (plain, roasted garlic, or roasted tomato)
4 large, low-carbohydrate tortillas
1 cup baby spinach
1 roasted pepper, cut into strips

Drain water from canned tuna or salmon and break into pieces. If using fresh tuna or salmon, brush olive oil on both sides of fish and sprinkle with herbs. Sauté in 1 teaspoon olive oil or bake at 350 degrees for 5–6 minutes until cooked to your preference. Fish should not be overcooked. Let fish stand to cool for about 5 minutes and slice.

Spread ¼ of hummus evenly over each tortilla and arrange ¼ of the spinach on top. Then place strips of roasted pepper on each. Finish with tuna or salmon. Roll wrap and serve immediately or wrap in plastic wrap and chill for later serving.

Makes 4 servings.

Turkey Chili

2 pounds ground turkey breast (or dark meat)
1 can (28 or 32 ounce can) tomatoes, undrained and cut up
2 cans (15 ounce cans) red kidney beans, drained
1 can (8 ounce can) tomato sauce
1 medium onion, chopped
¼–½ cup dry red wine, optional

2 tablespoons chili powder
1 teaspoon dried parsley flakes
¾ teaspoon dried basil, crushed
¾ teaspoon dried oregano, crushed
½ teaspoon black pepper
½ teaspoon ground cinnamon
1 clove garlic, minced
¼–½ teaspoon ground red pepper
1 bay leaf

In a 4-quart Dutch oven, brown the turkey for about 7–10 minutes. Drain fat. Stir in remaining ingredients and simmer uncovered for 45 minutes. Remove bay leaf before serving.

Makes 8 servings.

DESSERTS

Mango-Berry Meringue

5 cups fruit: any combination of berries, cherries, and/or mango
(my favorite is 3 cups sliced mango [about 3 mangos], fresh or frozen,
and 2 cups mixed frozen berries). Defrost if frozen.
¼ cup apple juice concentrate, defrosted
1 tablespoon lemon juice
1 tablespoon arrowroot or pectin
1 teaspoon vanilla extract
6 egg whites (large or extra-large eggs)

Combine fruit, apple juice concentrate, and lemon juice in a large saucepan. Bring to boil over medium heat. Reduce heat to a simmer, stirring constantly, for 3 minutes. Slowly stir in the pectin or arrowroot, and simmer for another 2–3 minutes until slightly thickened. Remove from heat and allow to cool for 15 minutes. Now preheat oven to 375 degrees.

In a medium bowl, beat egg whites until stiff peaks form. Carefully fold into the warm fruit, but do not over-mix. Pour mixture into a 13 x 9-inch baking dish and set the dish into a larger oven-proof pan. Pour boiling water into the larger pan about halfway up the sides of the baking dish. Bake for 20 minutes. Remove baking dish from the water and bake for another 2–3 minutes to brown the meringue slightly. Remove from oven and cool for 15 minutes before serving. It is also delicious when served chilled.

Makes 10–12 servings.

Gingerbread

½ cup pecans or walnuts, chopped finely

½ cup agave nectar or fruit sweetener
(concentrated peach, pineapple, and pear juice)

¼ cup canola oil

2 eggs or egg replacer

½ teaspoon grated orange rind

1 teaspoon vanilla extract

1½ cups brown rice flour or sorghum flour

½ teaspoon salt

1 teaspoon baking powder

1 teaspoon baking soda

2 teaspoons ground ginger

1½ teaspoons ground cinnamon

¼ teaspoon grated nutmeg

⅛ teaspoon cloves

1 cup unsweetened applesauce

In a large mixing bowl, combine the agave nectar or fruit sweetener and oil. Beat on high speed until thoroughly blended. Add the eggs, one at a time. Be sure to beat well after each addition. Add the orange rind and vanilla and continue to blend together. Set aside.

Preheat oven to 350 degrees and spray a 9-inch square pan with non-stick spray.

Sift together the dry ingredients and add the nuts.

Add some of the dry ingredients to the wet ingredients, a little at a time, blending well. Add ¼ cup of the applesauce, then blend. Add more dry mixture, and continue until you have combined all the ingredients.

Pour the batter into the pan and bake for 20–25 minutes or until gingerbread is done. Check for doneness by inserting a toothpick or touching lightly on the center. If the touch leaves an indent, the gingerbread is not done. If it springs back, remove to a cooling rack.

Note: Gingerbread freezes well.

Makes 9 servings.

Strawberry Sorbet
(adapted from *Gluten-free, Sugar-free Cooking,* by Sue O'Brien)

2 cups frozen strawberries

1 cup frozen blueberries

½ cup frozen orange juice concentrate

Place all ingredients in a blender and process until smooth. If mixture is too dry, add more orange juice concentrate. Garnish with a fresh berry or a sprig of mint.

You may substitute frozen pineapple, mango, or other juice.

Makes 4 servings.

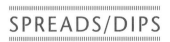

SPREADS/DIPS

White Bean Spread

You may use any mixture of light-colored beans, such as black-eyed peas, garbanzos, great northern, or white kidney beans (cannelloni)

2 cans (15 ounce cans) of above beans
¼ cup tahini (sesame nut butter)
¼ cup lemon juice
1 teaspoon lemon zest, optional
¼ cup extra-virgin olive oil
3 cloves garlic
1 tablespoon ground cumin
1 teaspoon cinnamon
1 teaspoon paprika
3 tablespoons tamari (low sodium soy sauce)

Put all ingredients in food processor and process until creamy. Add salt to taste as needed. Refrigerate or serve immediately with rye crackers or vegetable crudités, such as baby carrots, cucumber and celery sticks, fresh green beans or sugar snap peas, radishes, and cherry tomatoes. Use your imagination (broccoli or cauliflower florets or any veggies you like).

Makes 3 cups.

Endnotes

||||||||||||||||||||||||||||||||||||||||||||||||||||||||||||||||||||||

Chapter 1

1. *Textbook of Functional Medicine*, ed. David S. Jones and Sheila Quinn, 348 (Gig Harbor: WA: The Institute of Functional Medicine, 2006).

Chapter 3

1. D. E Nelson, et al., "State Trends in Health Risk Factors and Receipt of Clinical Preventive Services Among US Adults During the 1990s," *JAMA* 287:2659–2667.
2. W. Willett, *Eat, Drink and Be Healthy: The Harvard Medical School Guide to Healthy Eating* (New York: Simon and Schuster, 2001).
3. D. R. Kahn, "Triglycerides and Toggling the Tummy," *Nature Genetics* 25 (2000): 6–7.
4. J. S. Bland, "The Functional Medicine Approach to Treating Obesity," *International Journal of Integrative Medicine* 2 (November/December 2000): 37.
5. S. Lindeberg, L. Cordain, and S. B. Eaton, "Biological and Clinical Potential of a Paleolithic Diet," *Journal of Nutritional Environmental Medicine* 13 (2003):149–160.
6. R. M. Hackman, B. K. Ellis, and R. L. Brown, "Phosphorous Magnetic Resonance Spectra and Changes in Body Composition During Weight Loss," *J Am Coll Nutr* 13, 3 (1994): 243–250.
7. P. Kris-Etherton, R. H. Eckel, B. V. Howard, S. St. Jeor, and T. L. Bazzarre. "Lyon Diet Heart Study." *Circulation* 103 (2001): 1823.
8. K. Knoops, T. B. de Groot, et al., "Mediterranean Diet, Lifestyle Factors, and 10-Year Mortality in Elderly European Men and Women: the HALE Project," *JAMA* 292 (September 2004).

Chapter 4

1. J. S. Bland, "Functional Medicine Approach to Managing Syndrome X and Type 2 Diabetes," *International Journal of Integrative Medicine* 1 (November/December 1999):39–46.

2. C. Bogardus and G. Reaven, et al., "Relationship Between Degree of Obesity and in Vivo Insulin Action in the Man," *The American Journal of Physiology* 248 (1985):E286–E291.

3. O. E. Odeleye, M. de Courten, D. Pettitt, and E. Ravussin, "Fasting Hyperinsulinemia Is a Predictor of Increased Body Weight Gain and Obesity in Pima Indian Children," *Diabetes* 46 (1997):1341–1345.

4. J. V. Neel, "The 'Thrifty Genotype' in 1998," *Nutritional Review* 57 (1999):S2–S9.

5. N. Ruderman, D. Chisholm, X. Pi-Sunyer, and S. Schneider, "The Metabolically Obese, Normal-Weight Individual Revisited," *Diabetes* 47 (May 1998):704.

6. G. Reaven, *Syndrome X. Overcoming the Silent Killer That Can Give You a Heart Attack* (New York: Simon and Schuster, 2000).

7. M. L. Zoler, "Heart Association Advocates Fish Oil Supplements," *Family Practice News* (January 15, 2003):6.

8. A. Rivellese, A. Giacco, S. Genovese, et al., "Effect of Dietary Fibre on Blood Sugar Control and Serum Lipoproteins in Diabetic Patients," *Lancet* 2 (1980):447.

Chapter 5

1. Richard Shames, *Thyroid Power: Ten Steps to Total Health* (New York: Harper-Collins, 2001), p. 86.

2. R. Sapolsky, *Why Zebra Don't Get Ulcers: A Guide to Stress, Stress-Related Diseases, and Coping* (New York: W.H. Freeman & Co, 1998).

Chapter 6

1. S. O'Brien, *Gluten-free, Sugar-free Cooking* (New York: Marlowe & Co., 2005).

Chapter 7

1. Scott Rigden, *Functional Medicine Adjunctive Nutritional Support for CFS* (Gig Harbor, WA: Health Communications International, 1998).

Chapter 8

1. Scott Rigden, "An Analysis of Weight Loss Dropouts: The Ineffective Life-Style Syndrome," *The Bariatrician* (Summer 1989):22–30.

2. Scott Rigden, "The Ineffective Lifestyle Syndrome: A Bariatric Challenge," *The Bariatrician* (Summer 1995):8–13.

Glossary

||||||||||||||||||||||||||||||||||||||||||||||||||||||||||||||||||||||

acanthosis nigricans: This rash is often associated with metabolic syndrome. It is a dark pigmented rash (usually gray or brown) under the arms or breasts or on the back of the neck.

ACTH (adrenocorticotropic hormone): This is an adrenocorticotropic hormone that is released by the pituitary and stimulates the adrenal gland to release more cortisol, a key stress hormone.

adaptogenic medicinal plants: These are plants such as Panax ginseng, Siberian ginseng, Rhodiola crenulata, and Cordyceps sinensis that contain herbs that may enhance the body's anti-stress defense mechanisms.

adrenal glands: These glands are located on the kidneys. They are first-line responders to stress and release large amounts of cortisol and adrenaline-like hormones in response to stress.

aerobic exercise: Aerobic exercise involves the consumption of oxygen. These exercises are continuous and rhythmic, they improve the heart and lungs, and they stimulate fat burn-off. Examples are walking, jogging, biking, and swimming.

aldosterone: A hormone secreted by the adrenal gland that can affect sodium and fluid retention.

alopecia: Hair loss.

amenorrhea: Lack of menses.

arcus senilis: This abnormal finding in the eye is often associated with metabolic syndrome. Patients have a white arc or circle around the iris, which ordinarily should only be seen in much older patients.

asthma: An allergic disorder marked by difficulty in breathing, wheezing, and a cough.

bariatric medicine: The medical specialty that deals with the diagnosis and treatment of obesity and related medical and nutritional problems.

carbohydrate sensitivity: A tendency for some people to react to simple carbohydrates such as processed white bread, sugar, white potatoes, or refined grain cereals with an exaggerated release of sugar into the bloodstream after eating; this in turn provokes the body to release extra insulin to help the body to process the blood sugar.

Caveman/Cavewoman Diet: This diet was developed by Dr. Rigden. It is very effective for breaking insulin resistance and helping patients with metabolic syndrome. It is characterized by large amounts of healthy lean protein, heart-healthy fats, copious nonstarchy vegetables, and low-glycemic fruit.

CRH: Corticotropin-releasing hormone is released by the hypothalamus in response to stress; this hormone stimulates the pituitary to release ACTH.

CRP-hs: C-reactive protein, high sensitivity, is a coronary risk factor that measures the amount of inflammation in the coronary arteries. Inflammation is a problem because it accelerates hardening of the arteries. CRP-hs is often elevated in patients with metabolic syndrome.

cruciferous vegetables: These cabbage family vegetables include broccoli, Brussels sprouts, cabbage, cauliflower, bok choy, collards, kale, kohlrabi, mustard greens, radish, rutabaga, turnip, and watercress.

detox beverage: A hypoallergenic, rice-based protein formula containing selected nutrients that augment liver detoxification.

DHEA: Dihydroepiandrosterone is an important hormone secreted by the adrenal gland; it is often abnormal in PCOS patients.

eczema: An itching skin rash marked by oozing and then crusted lesions.

elimination diet: A diet that omits certain foods for 30 to 90 days that trigger food hypersensitivity reactions. The foods omitted can be those identified by RAST testing or they can be part of a standardized diet that is discussed in Chapter 6.

endocrine glands: Glands in the body that secrete hormonal substances into the bloodstream that can influence multiple areas of body functioning; examples are the thyroid and adrenal glands.

estrogen: The main female hormone secreted by females; typically there are three kinds of estrogen: estradiol, estrone, and estriol.

food hypersensitivity: An abnormal reaction of the immune system to certain trigger foods in the diet. This reaction involves excessive release of antibodies from the immune system that are usually provoked by microbes or pollens. These reactions can cause the release of toxins that can cause symptoms such headaches, skin rash, aches and pains, congestion, stomach problems, fluid retention, and weight gain.

functional medicine: A new field of medicine that employs nutrition and lifestyle assessment and interventions to improve physiological, emotional/cognitive, and physical function.

GALT: An acronym for gut-associated lymphoid tissue; 60 percent of the body's immune response comes from GALT.

genomics: The study of our genome, the sum of our 46 chromosomes, and the genes on these chromosomes; this gives information on how our DNA can be expressed in different ways to affect our body and health.

glycemic index: Measures the speed at which the body digests food, mainly carbohydrates, and converts it to blood sugar (glucose); the faster the food breaks down, the higher its rating on the index.

gout: A painful disorder of the joints, classically involving the foot and especially the large toe. It is very uncomfortable and is caused by elevated levels of uric acid that are deposited in the joints. Uric acid often is elevated in metabolic syndrome.

hirsutism: Unwanted facial hair in females. It is seen in metabolic syndrome and polycystic ovary syndrome (PCOS).

homocysteine: An inherited coronary risk factor in which the patient does not adequately convert the amino acid ornithine to cysteine. The aberrant amino acid produced, homocysteine, can be an abrasive to the inner lining of the arteries, making them more prone to forming plaque. Supplements of B-6, B-12, and folic acid can be helpful in normalizing this situation.

HRT: Stands for hormone replacement therapy, used for perimenopausal or menopausal females; this can be done with pharmaceuticals or natural bio-identical hormones.

hyperinsulinemia: Refers to having excessive levels of insulin in the bloodstream. Insulin not only regulates blood sugar, it also regulates fat storage. Therefore, hyperinsulinemia tends to promote fat storage and obesity.

hyperlipidemia: Excess fats (or lipids) in the bloodstream such as cholesterol and triglycerides.

IgE antibodies (immunoglobulins): Proteins usually released by the immune system to protect the body from allergens such as pollen or insect stings.

IgG antibodies (immunoglobulins): Proteins usually released by the immune system to protect the body from microbes.

indole-3-carbinol: Nutrient found in cruciferous vegetables that influence estrogen metabolism.

infertility: The inability to conceive.

inflammatory cytokines: Disruptive, toxic chemicals that cause pain, swelling, redness, or itching. In the context of this chapter, they can be released in response to a reaction of IgG antibodies to food break-down particles in the bloodstream.

insulin resistance: The insulin in the body secreted by the pancreas is not as effective as it should be. Even though the levels of insulin may actually be elevated, people with insulin resistance cannot utilize the insulin. This leads to the pancreas trying to compensate by releasing more and more insulin, which can lead to very negative health consequences like obesity and diabetes.

irritable bowel syndrome: A disorder of the colon that is characterized by abnormal elimination patterns; these can be marked by loose, urgent, frequent stools, diarrhea, gas, bloating, and constipation. Sometimes there is alternating diarrhea and constipation.

isometric exercise: Resistance exercises that increase strength and tone muscles. These exercises include weight-lifting, either with free weights or using weight machines, or exercises that use the weight of the body for resistance.

leaky gut syndrome: A gut condition characterized by increased intestinal permeability, which occurs when the wall of the small intestine is damaged. This permeability allows toxins made by bacteria, yeast, and/or parasites to leak out of the gut into systemic circulation, where they can cause symptoms of inflammation, compromise the immune system, and impair liver detoxification. In addition, large molecules of partially digested foods can escape from a permeable gut.

LH/FSH: Hormones released by the pituitary gland that are often abnormal in PCOS patients. LH stands for luteinizing hormone and FSH stands for follicle-stimulating hormone.

liver detoxification: The process by which the liver protects us from toxins in the environment and in our diet that circulate throughout our bloodstream. These toxins come from our food, water, and air; on a more subtle level, these toxins can originate from toxins manufactured in our bodies, microbes, and prescription drugs.

medical food for insulin management: A nutritional supplement specifically developed to support individuals with insulin resistance and hyperinsulinemia (too much insulin). It is a soy-based protein powder that is low-glycemic and contains high-amylose starch. In contrast to typical starches in the diet, it is slowly broken down and released from the stomach into the bloodstream gradually after ingestion. This leads to a long, slow release of blood sugar, smoothing out the patient's blood sugar and insulin response.

Mediterranean diet: This is a very healthy diet, much studied by researchers, that is consumed by the inhabitants of southern France,

Italy, Greece, and other countries in the Mediterranean region. It is associated with longevity, very little obesity, and far less diabetes and heart disease than we see in the United States. It is characterized by the consumption of relatively large amounts of vegetables and fruit, heart-healthy fats, and low glycemic dietary choices in general.

menopause/perimenopause: Menopause refers to total cessation of menstrual cycles in the female; perimenopause refers to the period of time between normal menstrual cycles and menopause, often defined by irregular menses, spotting, and/or heavy menstrual flow.

metabolic syndrome: A common cause of obesity in people with the apple-shaped body type; too much insulin in the body, which is not effective because of insulin resistance, characterizes it. These overweight people often have borderline blood sugar, high blood pressure, high triglycerides, and low HDL, and they are generally pre-diabetic.

metabolism: The process by which food substances are handled in the body. In this book, metabolism particularly refers to the body's ability to efficiently break down food for energy (efficient metabolism) and other necessary bodily processes versus its tendency to store the calories from food (sluggish or slow metabolism).

micronutrients: Nutritional factors in the body like vitamins and minerals that are needed in very small amounts for healthy cellular functioning and metabolism; often they are deficient in patients with metabolic syndrome and these deficiencies are associated with increased metabolic problems. They can be given as supplements and can be an effective part of a program to normalize metabolic syndrome.

nutriceuticals: Natural supplements developed to have specific physiological and/or pharmacological effects to help the body to achieve health.

nutrigenomics: The study of how different foods may interact with specific genes to modify the risk of common, chronic diseases like diabetes and obesity.

paleolithic diet: The type of basic, low glycemic diet eaten by our ancestors in the Stone Age (paleolithic period).

phytoestrogens: Naturally occurring plant nutrients that cause mild estrogen-like activity in the body; examples are isoflavones in soy and lignans in flaxseed.

PMS: Premenstrual syndrome. Symptoms are weight gain, bloating, and irritability that occur in susceptible females three to seven days prior to menses.

polycystic ovary syndrome (PCOS): This condition affects 6 to 10 percent of women of reproductive age. It is the most common cause of anovulatory infertility, in which females have menstrual cycles without ovulation. Seventy percent of PCOS women are obese. Elevated levels of androgen, ovulation problems, and ovarian cysts define this condition.

progesterone: A female hormone secreted when ovulation occurs.

RAST test: A blood test that is able to detect increased levels of IgG and/or IgE antibodies that the body has released in response to a trigger food.

skin tags: Often associated with metabolic syndrome, these are small growths located around the neck and upper body.

sleep apnea: A sleep disorder, often associated with metabolic syndrome; it is characterized by erratic breathing, often associated with snoring, that compromises oxygenation of the brain during the night. The following day often is characterized by fatigue and sleepiness.

SPPMRP: The Soy Protein Powder Meal Replacement Program is an extremely successful program for patients with carbohydrate sensitivity. In essence, it involves two soy protein meal replacements, two to three low-glycemic snacks, and one low-glycemic meal. The soy protein powder is a very high quality, low-glycemic product that provides excellent levels of protein, vitamins, and minerals.

switched metabolism: An impaired metabolism in which the person's body is preferentially storing calories consumed in the diet as fat for that proverbial "rainy day."

Synthroid: A common prescription of T4 (thyroxine).

systolic and diastolic blood pressure: The top number of the blood pressure 120/80 reading is the systolic blood pressure. It is the pressure in your arteries when your heart is beating. The bottom number is the diastolic pressure, the pressure in your arteries when your heart is resting between beats. So, in this example, 120 is the systolic blood pressure and 80 is the diastolic blood pressure.

target heart rate: Maximum heart rate is the number of times per minute your heart pumps when it is working at 100 percent capacity. Never exercise at your maximum heart rate. Knowing your maximum heart rate will help you calculate your target heart rate, the number of beats per minute your heart should pump during aerobic exercise. In general, if you are relatively fit, your target heart rate should be 70 to 85 percent of your maximum heart rate. However, if you are in a poor state of fitness and more than 20 pounds overweight, your initial target heart rate should be 60 to 70 percent of your maximum heart rate. Reaching your target heart rate indicates your body is receiving maximum cardiovascular and fat-burning benefits.

testosterone: The main androgenic hormone in females; it is often abnormally high in females with PCOS.

T4, T3: The thyroid gland releases T4 (thyroxine), which circulates in the bloodstream and attaches to receptors in many organs of the body. Some of T4 is transformed to T3 in the liver; T3 is very important for burning fat.

thyroid gland: A gland located at the base of the neck that is a key player in weight loss metabolism and the production of physical energy.

triglycerides: A type of fat circulating in the bloodstream that is derived from fatty acids made by the liver in response to the intake of blood sugar. These can, in some cases, become excessive and contribute to blockages in the blood vessels.

TSH: Stands for thyroid stimulating hormone, which is released from the pituitary to stimulate the thyroid to release thyroid hormone; it is also measured in the most commonly measured lab test to determine if the thyroid is over or underactive.

xenobiotics: Chemical substances that are foreign, and usually harmful, to the organism (e.g., PCPs).

Resources

|||||||||||||||||||||||||||||||||||||||||||||||||||||||||||||||||||||||||||||

Books

Baker, Sidney. *Detoxification and Healing*. New Canaan, CT: Keats Publishing, 1997.

Bland, Jeffrey. *Genetic Nutritioneering*. Los Angeles, CA: Keats Publishing, 1998.

Brand-Miller, Jennie, and Kaye Foster Powell. *The New Glucose Revolution Shopper's Guide to GI Values 2007: The Authoritative Source of Glycemic Index Values for More Than 500 Foods*. New York: Marlowe and Co., 2006.

Foreyt, John. *Living without Dieting*. New York: Time Warner, 1997.

Galland, Leo. *The Four Pillars of Healing*. New York: Random House, 1997.

Gallop, Rick. *The GI Diet*. Ontario, Canada: Random House Canada, 2002.

Jones, David. *Healthy Changes*. Ashland, OR: HealthComm, 2000.

Katzen, Mollie, and Walter Willett. *Eat, Drink, and Weigh Less*. New York: Hyperion, 2006.

O'Brien, Susan. *Gluten-free Sugar-free Cooking: Over 200 Delicious Recipes to Help You Live a Healthier, Allergy-Free Life*. New York: Marlowe and Company, 2006.

Reaven, Gerald. *Syndrome X: Overcoming the Silent Killer that Can Give You a Heart Attack*. New York: Simon-Schuster, 2002.

Segersten, Alissa, and Tom Malterre. *The Whole Life Nutrition Cookbook*, 2nd ed. Bellingham, WA: Whole Life Press, 2006.

Textbook of Functional Medicine, edited by David S. Jones and Sheila Quinn. Gig Harbor, WA: Institute of Functional Medicine, 2005.

Wansink, Brian. *Mindless Eating*. New York: Bantam Books, 2007.

Willett, Walter, and P. J. Skerrett. *Eat, Drink, and Be Healthy: The Harvard Medical School Guide To Healthy Eating*. New York: Free Press, 2005.

Other Resources

Living Without: A Lifestyle Guide for People with Allergies and Food Sensitivities. This is a wonderful magazine for those with food allergies. You can sign up for a weekly recipe at www.livingwithout.com that is sent via e-newsletter.

Weight-Control Information Network
Email: WIN@info.niddk.nih.gov
Website: www.niddk.nih.gov/health/nutrit/nutrit.htm
The Weight-control Information Network (WIN) is a service of the National Institute of Diabetes and Digestive and Kidney Diseases of the National Institutes of Health

Food and Nutrition Information Center, U.S. Dept. of Agriculture
Website: www.nal.usda.gov/fnic

Index

More Hunter House Books

IT AIN'T OVER 'TIL THE THIN LADY SINGS: How to Make Your Weight Loss Surgery a Lasting Success by Michelle Ritchie, CSAC, ICRC

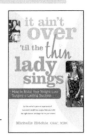

In this book the author shares her knowledge as a weight-loss-surgery group facilitator, discusses her life before and after surgery, and explains why she chose to have the operation. Ritchie reveals how obesity kept her from enjoying "normal" activities, applying for jobs, or having an active sex life. She emphasizes that surgery is not a quick-fix solution but a tool, and highlights the importance of the choices the patient makes after the procedure. Her book includes:

* a detailed description of gastric bypass surgery and how it works
* tools for assessing whether weight loss surgery is right for you and tips for keeping weight off after surgery
* guides for identifying "trigger foods" and making better food choices
* a daily food plan for post-op patients, sample shopping lists, and a chart of amino acid supplements to help stave off cravings
* information on how to approach intimacy and relationships after surgery

256 pages ... 2 Illus. ... 5 b/w photos ... Paperback $15.95

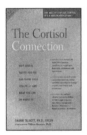

THE CORTISOL CONNECTION: Why Stress Makes You Fat and Ruins Your Health — and What You Can Do About It by Shawn Talbott, PhD

Cortisol is the body's main stress hormone, triggering our fight-or-flight reactions when we deal with stressful situations. Prolonged stress causes the body's cortisol levels to rise, and research has shown that high cortisol levels are associated with obesity, diabetes, and even Alzheimer's disease.

In the first edition of this book, Talbott introduced his SENSE program that showed readers how to manage stress and reduce cortisol levels. In the second edition the program has been refined with new research and five years of testing. Talbott also describes the connection between cortisol and HSD and cortisol and testosterone which, if kept within normal ranges, help us to maximize the metabolic effect of diet and exercise regimens — and improve weight loss.

336 pages ... 7 illus. ... 21 tables ... Paperback $15.95 ... 2nd Edition

THE CORTISOL CONNECTION DIET: The Breakthrough Program to Control Stress and Lose Weight by Shawn Talbott, PhD

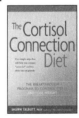

The stress hormone cortisol is a key factor in obesity and cortisol control is the missing link in effective weight loss. Higher cortisol levels increase appetite, enhance fat storage, and disrupt blood sugar control. In *The Cortisol Connection Diet,* Shawn Talbott shows how to apply the research descibed in *The Cortisol Connection.* This pocket-sized guide

* explains how to use food, dietary supplements, and exercise to control cortisol and blood sugar levels
* shows you how to change your metabolic response to food, essential for losing those last 10 pounds.

Included are a three-week log to chart diet, exercise and supplements, and sample plans for breakfast, lunch, dinner, snacks and supplements.

144 pages ... 5 illus. ... 7 tables ... 7 charts ... Paperback $9.95

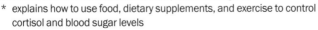

More Hunter House Books

THE ANTI-INFLAMMATION DIET AND RECIPE BOOK: Protect Your-self and Your Family from Heart Disease, Arthritis, Diabetes, Allergies —and More by Jessica K. Black, ND

Jessica Black wrote this book for patients who were trying to follow a naturo-pathic, anti-inflammatory diet. She prepared and tested all the recipes her-self, using organic and nutrient-rich foods, eliminating common allergenic foods, and reducing the intake of pesticides and hormones — all of which help to build a stronger, healthier, healing body.

The first part of the book explains how the anti-inflammation diet works. The second part contains 125 simple and tasty recipes, from breakfasts, appetiz-ers and herbal teas to soups, entrees, salads, and delicious desserts. Most of the recipes take little time to fix, and include substitution suggestions and health tips. Sample eating plans are included for the summer and winter months, so you can get the added benefit of eating what's in season.

256 pages ... Paperback $15.95 ... Spiralbound $19.95

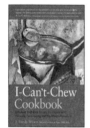

I-CAN'T-CHEW COOKBOOK: Delicious Soft-Diet Recipes for People with Chewing, Swallowing and Dry-Mouth Disorders by J. Randy Wilson

Over 40 million people in the U.S. have chewing and swallowing disorders, caused by surgery, mouth/throat cancer, TMJ problems, braces or den-tures, stroke, Alzheimer's, AIDS, or lupus. Often, they exist on milkshakes, Jell-O, mashed potatoes, and baby food. This book explains how they can get the real food their body needs to recover from surgery and disease.

This is not a liquid diet book or a blender cookbook: Inside are over 150 recipes for tasty casseroles, soups, and main dishes featuring crab, salmon, ham, and chicken. There are Mexican-flavored entrées, vegetables that are chopped not puréed, and great desserts — food the whole family can enjoy. Each recipe comes with a complete nutritional analysis, so that you can be sure your meals are healthy and nutritionally sound. Also available in a lie-flat spiral binding.

224 pages ... Paperback $16.95 ... Spiralbound $22.95

THE *NATURAL* ESTROGEN DIET & RECIPE BOOK
by Lana Liew, MD, and Linda Ojeda, PhD

This book is the answer for women who are concerned about the poten-tially negative effects of hormome replacement therapy (HRT) and are look-ing for safe, effective, and natural ways to reduce their menopausal and postmenopausal symptoms. The book is divided into two parts. **Part One** discusses up-to-date research findings relevant to women's health as well as information on phytoestrogens (plant estrogens) and how they can alle-viate the symptoms of menopause and promote a woman's health. **Part Two** provides over 100 recipes the whole family can enjoy. Chapters include

* Integrating Natural Estrogens into Your Life
* Appetizers, Snacks, and Pick-Me-Ups
* Salads, Side Dishes, and Main Courses
* Pancakes, Breads, Muffins, and Desserts

Includes a glossary and resource section, and a nutritional analysis of all recipes.

256 pages ... Paperback $14.95 ... 2nd Edition

More Hunter House Books

THE NO-BEACH, NO-ZONE, NO-NONSENSE WEIGHT-LOSS PLAN:
A Pocket Guide to What Works *by Jim Johnson, PT*

The No-Beach, No-Zone, No-Nonsense Weight-Loss Plan is based on a "what works" analysis of studies on weight loss. The author has identified the strategies that really work — and can be done at home. He explains
* how to determine your body mass index (BMI) and calorie needs
* whether your weight is threatening your health and why your weight problem may not be all your fault
* how to calculate the percentage of fats, carbohydrates, and protein in your diet

Complete with exercise and calorie-count cards, *The No-Beach, No-Zone, No-Nonsense Weight-Loss Plan* is for everyone. It will appeal to dieters who have tried plans that haven't worked, parents who want to start overweight children on a non-fad approach, and doctors, nurses, and other health-care professionals.

144 pages ... 6 illus. ... 7 tables ... Paperback $8.95

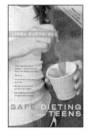

SAFE DIETING FOR TEENS *by Linda Ojeda, PhD*

Teens today live in an image-conscious society where they are confronted with weight issues every day. Many resort to skipping meals, taking laxatives, or throwing up after eating. But there is a much safer and more effective way to get fit and trim. In *Safe Dieting for Teens,* Linda Ojeda, a certified nutritionist, combines personal insights and professional expertise to offer teens the knowledge they need to create their own diet program. No food is off limits, so teens can adapt the information to their own choices and goals. This book explains
* the math of losing weight, the benefits of exercise, and how to select the right foods at the right time
* girls' special diet dilemma and healthy alternatives for meals, snacks, and drinks
* the dangers of bad dieting, how to spot a dangerous diet program, and the pros and cons of popular diets such as low-carb and Jenny Craig.

168 pages ... Paperback $14.95 ... 2nd Edition

AWESOME FOODS FOR ACTIVE KIDS: The ABCs of Eating for
Energy and Health *by Anita Bean, BSc*

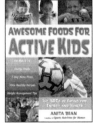

This practical guide contains all the information and suggestions you need to feed growing kids, from kindergarten through high school. Beginning with the basics of children's nutrition, Anita Bean explains how to incorporate the best nutrients into your child's diet, how much of each nutrient your child needs, and where they can get it from. Special chapters address the needs of athletes, fussy eaters, overweight children, and eating at school. By building their bodies with nutrients now, your children can grow into healthy, active adults. Includes answers to questions like:
* How do I feed my vegetarian child?   * How much fat should my child have?
* How can I keep my athlete hydrated?   * What should they eat after exercise?
... and much, much more.

224 pages ... 29 b/w photos ... 49 illus. ... 32 tables ... 87 recipes ... Paperback $16.95

More Hunter House Books

THE IBS HEALING PLAN: Natural Ways to Beat Your Symptoms
by Theresa Cheung

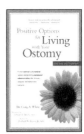

Irritable bowel syndrome (IBS) affects 15–20 percent of adults in the U.S. yet, all too often, people affected by IBS choose to suffer in silence. Theresa Cheung's book, packed full of information and help for those suffering from the abdominal pain, bloating, and irregular bowel habits that are the symptoms of IBS, clearly explains the causes and symptoms.

The healing plan focuses on five key areas: diet, supplements, complementary therapies, stress management, and working with your doctor. Natural remedies include yoga, acupuncture, supplements, stress management, and dietary changes. There is also detailed information about over-the-counter and prescription drugs, their benefits, and their drawbacks.

Clearly written and easy to navigate, this book is useful for sufferers, doctors, and friends and family alike.

168 pages ... 9 illus. ... Paperback $14.95

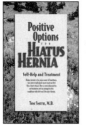

POSITIVE OPTIONS FOR HIATUS HERNIA: Self-Help and Treatment
by Tom Smith, MD

A hiatus hernia is a common and potentially serious condition that occurs when the upper part of the stomach pushes through the diaphragm, causing a gastric reflux condition that is the source of chronic pain for 30 percent of American adults. This book describes how a hiatus hernia comes about, why it could be dangerous, and how to protect yourself from more serious developments including esophageal cancer. It includes information on:

* tests and medical treatments, including the latest drug and surgery options
* self-help, including diet, eating habits, basic fitness, and stress management

The clear information will help you to get the treatments and make lifestyle changes you need to manage this poorly recognized but widespread condition and live free of symptoms.

128 pages ... 4 illus. ... Paperback $12.95

POSITIVE OPTIONS FOR LIVING WITH YOUR OSTOMY: Self-Help and Treatment *by Dr. Craig A. White*

An ostomy is a surgically created opening used to expel waste when the body's normal systems are damaged. This book provides the information you need to deal with the practical and emotional aspects of life after ostomy surgery. Dr. White describes what happens before and during the surgery; how to adapt to wearing an ostomy-care appliance, and how to care for and change it.

Aware of the long-term concerns of patients and their families, Dr. White provides extensive information on recognizing common emotional reactions, including anxiety and depression, adapting proactively, and knowing when to seek help. Helpful lists and forms provide guidelines for dealing with changes in social interactions, intimate relationships, and sexual activity.

144 pages ... 4 illus. ... Paperback $12.95